"*An At-Home Guide to Children's Sensory and Behavioral Pr.* wonderful introduction to the Qigong method of soothing ch..... .... Garofallou and Silva have written a remarkable book about the remarkable power of touch for physical, emotional, cognitive, social and prosocial development. All parents – indeed, all of us – will benefit from reading this *tour de force*."

Stuart Shanker, DPhil, *distinguished Research Professor Emeritus of philosophy and psychology; Founder of the MEHRIT Centre, Ltd., and Self-Reg Global Inc.*

"Touch, sensory processing and self-regulation are central to every child's development. This book is bursting with richly detailed, yet clear and simple explanations of how these three key neurosensory domains work. It shows parents and clinicians how they can use touch to help children whose behavior says they need help to process their sensory experiences and regulate themselves. Parents and clinicians will also find here a similar approach – to give themselves the support they need to support their children's growth and healing."

Joshua Sparrow, MD, *Brazelton Touchpoints Center, Boston Children's Hospital/Harvard Medical School.*

"*An At-Home Guide to Children's Sensory and Behavioral Problems* weds Eastern and Western traditions of soma and psyche into a seamless hands-on book to promote the optimal development of self-regulation in children through sensory co-regulation and emotionally attuned parenting. Illuminating and practical, this conceptually sound and functional book is a must have for parents and professionals alike."

Gilbert M. Foley, EdD, IMH-E, *co-author*, Linking Sensory Integration and Mental Health: Nurturing Self-Regulation in Infants and Young Children *and* Mental Health in Early Intervention.

"As a developmental behavioral pediatrician with over 25 years caring for families who have children with autism spectrum disorders, I am very excited to recommend Qigong Sensory Treatment for Parents & Clinicians: An At-Home Guide to Children's Sensory and Behavioral Problems. This approach to therapeutic touch offers a new (and very ancient!) way to help children regulate not only their sensory systems; QST can have a real impact on the children's emotional, physical, and behavioral self-regulation issues including sleep problems, tantrums, stomach upsets and even aggression. The book is nicely organized with many detailed helpful and practical suggestions for making QST soothing and enjoyable for the children. QST will be a welcome complement to more traditional behavioral and developmental interventions."

Richard Solomon MD, FAAP, *author of* Autism: The Potential Within; *Medical Director, The PLAY Project*

An At-Home Guide to Children's Sensory and Behavioral Problems

An At-Home Guide to Children's Sensory and Behavioral Problems gives a new perspective on sensory and behavior problems, one that sees those behaviors as stemming from a child's immature sensory nervous system and regulation difficulties.

This book offers an effective at-home intervention, the Qigong Sensory Treatment, that enlists a parent's attuned touch to address often-overlooked sensory issues that underlie 'problem' behaviors and works to organize those sensory experiences to foster connection and the capacity for self-regulation. It introduces the reader to a new and clinically useful model to understand sensory development, the Early Childhood Self-regulatory Milestones which are critical to the emotional and behavioral health and regulation for all children. With clear step-by-step instructions, diagrams, and links to online instructional videos, it teaches parents how to successfully implement the daily QST hands-on routine.

Unique to the treatment model is how it guides and focuses parents to easily recognize, interpret and respond to their child's shifting non-verbal body and behavioral responses and cues. An extensive workbook section navigates parents through a year-long process of learning and implementing QST at home. Weekly letters include those written by the authors, parents who share their own personal experiences and by QST Master Trainers who offer their years of experience and helpful tips. The 52 letters are timed to anticipate and answer typical questions or stumbling blocks that parents commonly encounter at key points, guiding them to success with their child's sensory and behavior difficulties while making for happier and less stressful times with their child.

This guide will be indispensable to parents and clinicians looking to understand and more effectively work with their child's developmental difficulties.

Linda Garofallou, MS, QST Trainer, Adjunct Faculty at the Center for Autism & Early Childhood Mental Health/Montclair State University, has developed a wide range of community pediatric sensory programs for at risk children, including 14 years at Children's Hospital of NJ/Newark Beth Israel Medical Center.

Louisa Silva, MD, MPH, Pediatrician integrating Western and Chinese medicine with public health. Founder of Qigong Sensory Training Institute. Lead Researcher of 20 university based QST research studies for children with autism and other disabilities. Founder of the Guadalupe Community Clinic, Salem, OR.

An At-Home Guide to Children's Sensory and Behavioral Problems

Qigong Sensory Treatment for Parents and Clinicians

Linda Garofallou, MS
and Louisa Silva, MD, MPH

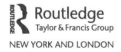

Routledge
Taylor & Francis Group

NEW YORK AND LONDON

QSTI Non-Profit Status

The Qigong Sensory Training Institute (QSTI) is a registered non-profit corporation dedicated to furthering education and research in Qigong Sensory Treatment for children with developmental disabilities. A portion of the proceeds from the sale of this book will go to the Qigong Sensory Training Institute. QSTI and related logos are trademarks belonging to the Qigong Sensory Training Institute. [www.QSTI.org]

Cover image: © Getty Images

First published 2024
by Routledge
605 Third Avenue, New York, NY 10158

and by Routledge
4 Park Square, Milton Park, Abingdon, Oxon, OX14 4RN

Routledge is an imprint of the Taylor & Francis Group, an informa business

Library of Congress Cataloging-in-Publication Data
Names: Garofallou, Linda, author. | Silva, Louisa, author.
Title: An at-home guide to children's sensory and behavioral problems : Qigong Sensory Treatment for parents and clinicians / by Linda Garofallou and Louisa Silva, MD, MPH.
Description: New York, NY : Routledge, 2024. | Includes bibliographical references and index.
Identifiers: LCCN 2023016114 (print) | LCCN 2023016115 (ebook) | ISBN 9781032419299 (paperback) | ISBN 9781003360421 (ebook)
Subjects: LCSH: Sensory integration dysfunction in children—Physical therapy. | Qi gong—Therapeutic use. | Massage for children.
Classification: LCC RJ496.S44 G37 2024 (print) | LCC RJ496.S44 (ebook) | DDC 618.92/8—dc23/eng/20230628
LC record available at https://lccn.loc.gov/2023016114
LC ebook record available at https://lccn.loc.gov/2023016115

ISBN: 978-1-032-41929-9 (pbk)
ISBN: 978-1-003-36042-1 (ebk)

DOI: 10.4324/9781003360421

Typeset in Times New Roman
by Apex CoVantage, LLC

Access the Support Material: https://resourcecentre.routledge.com/books/9781032419299

Contents

A Note on Vocabulary   *xiii*
Foreword   *xiv*
Preface and Acknowledgments   *xviii*

Welcome to QST!   1

PART I
Pulling Back the Curtain   11

  1 Behavior Through a Sensory Lens   13

  2 Self-Regulation – A Parent's Gift   21

  3 Attuned Touch – Your Sensory Solution   27

  4 QST – A Sensory Language   35

  5 Attuned Connections and Safe Boundaries   41

  6 The Key Ingredient – You   47

PART II
Learning QST at Home   53

  7 Getting Started   55

  8 Qigong Sensory Treatment: Step-by-Step Instructions   63

  9 Reading Your Child's Body Language   90

  10 How to Work Through the Difficult Spots   98

11 QST for Everyday 'Challenging' Behaviors   103

12 Optimizing Diet, Nutrition and Daily Routines   112

PART III
Guiding Your Way With 52 Weekly Letters   123

   Introduction to Weekly Letters   125

   Mastering the Basics – Weeks 1–14   127
    Week 1   Patting or Pressing – Learning What Works Best 127
    Week 2   Parent Self-Care and Self-Compassion 128
    Week 3   Getting Started 129
    Week 4   Working With Resistance to Touch 131
    Week 5   Lending Your Calm 132
    Week 6   Attuning to Your Child's Energy Level to Bring Calm 133
    Week 7   Pain and Ticklishness 135
    Week 8   Numbness 136
    Week 9   Signs QST is Working 137
    Week 10 More Signs QST is Working 139
    Week 11 Opening Roadblocks to Development 140
    Week 12 Persisting Through Frustrating and Difficult Times 141
    Week 13 Getting Comfortable and Noticing More 143
    Week 14 Widening the Circle of QST Helpers 144

   QST for Daily Regulation – Weeks 15–20   147
    Week 15 QST to Support Emotional Regulation 147
    Week 16 Sleep Problems 148
    Week 17 Listening Problems 149
    Week 18 Tantrums 150
    Week 19 Regulating Digestion and Elimination 152
    *Week 20 Reading Body and Behavioral Cues – Perspectives From Chinese
                 Medicine 153*

   Staying Consistent – Weeks 21–25   155
    Week 21 Making it Through the 'Dog Days' 155
    Week 22 The Four Risk Periods for Dropping the Daily QST Routine 156
    Week 23 Staying the Course 158
    Week 24 A Skeptical Parent Comes to Believe 159
    Week 25 Still Hyper? Diet is Key 160

Noticing Changes – Marking Progress – Weeks 26–32   161

Week 26   Noticing Changes and Progress Over Time 161
Week 27   Mid-Year Check-In 162
Week 28   Checking in on Your Goals 169
Week 29   Changes and What They Mean 170
Week 30   "Ready to Learn" 171
Week 31   Doing QST 6–7 Days A Week Versus 3–4 Days 172
Week 32   A Last Resort 173

Extra Techniques – Weeks 33–42   175

Week 33   A Simple Technique to Stop Aggressive Behavior 175
Week 34   Getting Your Child out of Defense Mode 177
Week 35   Points From Chinese Medicine That Help the Brain 178
Week 36   The Easy Button 179
Week 37   The Face-Me Button 180
Week 38   Making Transitions Easier 181
Week 39   Adapting to My Child's Needs 182
Week 40   Release of Emotions During QST 183
Week 41   Emotional Bubbles – How to Help 184
Week 42   Getting Through Emotionally Hard Times 185

QST for Specific Needs – Weeks 43–50   187

Week 43   Stuck in Stress Mode 187
Week 44   Reframing the Need for Control 188
Week 45   What to Do About Regression 189
*Week 46   Widening Social Circles (Parents – Siblings – Grandparents –
           Friends) 191*
Week 47   Sensory Problems and Success in School 192
Week 48   Unlocking My Child's Potential 193
Week 49   QST for the Home Medicine Cabinet 194
Week 50   The Importance of Early Self-Regulation for Adulthood 195

Year's End – Weeks 51–52   196

Week 51   Year-End Evaluation 196
Week 52   Final Thoughts and Appreciations 202

Appendix A QST Sensory Movement Chart and Guiding Tips   203
Appendix B Troubleshooting Guide   206
Appendix C Contraindications to the QST Sensory Protocol   210
Appendix D Getting Personalized QST Help   211

Appendix E Creating a Local QST Parent Support Group   *212*
Appendix F QST in Early Intervention   *214*
Appendix G Lessons Learned From QST Autism Research   *217*
Appendix H Accessing Online QST Support Materials   *221*
Index   *222*

A Note on Vocabulary

We live in a world rich in definitions of "family". In writing this book, we refer to the primary caregiver as "parent" and the second adult most connected to the child as "parent" or "partner". We see in these words, the connection that is unique to children and the particular adult(s) who, in the parental role, shelter, love, nourish and teach them. A parent or caregiver who is the only adult in the household should not despair. A second adult is helpful, but absolutely not required. Also, while we appreciate and celebrate the growing acknowledgement of unique individual identities in our language, to ensure ease of readability and clarity, we have decided to use only a single pronoun consistently throughout each chapter or segment, alternating that usage ("she" or "he") from chapter to chapter.

Foreword

In the beginning there is the relationship, and the relationship begins with touch! The power of relationships has emerged as the single most influential force in our unfolding as human beings. Our bodies and brains are relationally organized! For the authors, relationship is understood and communicated through the most basic of sensory modalities, touch. Human touch sits at the heart of this book. From that elemental and very human origin, Garofallou and Silva offer a novel, at-home, touch-based intervention founded on a deep understanding of touch's direct links to the brain and its critical role in the organization of sensory experience and, ultimately, in behavior and self-regulation itself. The sweep is wide and deep, but readers will find themselves immersed in a rich story, supported by a wealth of examples and resources giving parents real-time guidance that is clearly expressed and easy to understand.

For both the parent and the practitioner, there are few books that will be as transformational about the ways you think about and understand the meaning of human behavior, especially what you have come to think of as early childhood misbehavior. The authors see those (mis)behaviors as rooted in often-overlooked underlying sensory and self-regulation problems and the treatment and resolution as rooted in the relationship, mediated by organized loving touch itself. And that leads them and the reader to two innovative conclusions. First, it places the parent or primary caregiver at the heart of the therapeutic process. In fact, while this book is written for parents and clinicians, it is the parent who delivers the primary mode of treatment, and the book fully prepares parents for that process. While that preparation includes step-by-step instructions, self-exploration and (as I will illustrate below) new perspectives on their sensory child's inner state, it also offers something more, something unique – though designed as a treatment, QST was fundamentally conceived of as a two-person communication, one that builds healthier sensory pathways and strengthens the capacity for self-regulation.

And it is here that the authors offer their most valuable contribution. The reader is presented with what amounts to a Rosetta Stone by which to comprehend and speak to their sensory child *through sensory channels*. To achieve this, Garofallou and Silva spell out in clear and simple terms how touch forms the basis of a living 'sensory language' by which the parent or clinician can convey what is therapeutic and organizing to the overwhelmed child. And with it, a sensory child can be 'spoken to' and 'listened to' at the preverbal and pre-symbolic level. This is the level where real therapeutic action can occur. It is also a level that, in our current therapeutics, we too often tend to forget in favor of too much language.

I have known Linda Garofallou for nearly 25 years, and I have known of her work with Dr. Louisa Silva for over a decade. I have been privileged to learn from Linda as she pulls back the curtain on behavior and therapeutics. Old dichotomies fade away. Distinctions, like biological versus psychological (or body vs. mind) and development versus learning, appear artificial and misleading. Approaches to 'misbehavior' that emerge from longstanding and fading paradigms are reframed. What you have seen and understood for many years of parenting and practice will be reconsidered through a new set of eyes. As you will read in this book, "if you see a child differently, you see a different child" (Shanker & Barker, 2016).

This shift in your understanding will create disequilibrium in you – an imbalance that will lead you to deep questioning and even resistance as you are forced to reframe familiar behaviors in new ways. You will be rewarded for this imbalance with growth in understanding and practice. This will challenge all approaches that focus on manifest behavior – the 'back-end' – by instead framing behaviors as effectively communicating the origins of that behavior – the 'front-end'. You will reframe developmental and behavioral challenges in many instances as sensory difficulties. And you will learn to speak to those sensory difficulties through the 'language' of the new sensory communication that is QST.

Each chapter carefully builds on your understanding of the inextricable connections among our sensory systems and how these 'energies' lead to behaviors. Stuart Shanker (2016) urged all to reframe 'misbehavior' as 'stress behavior'. Garofallou and Silva further that process by helping the reader reframe 'misbehavior' as attempts by the child to adapt – as intuitive efforts at escaping the disorganization, distress and suffering from a nervous system that is not working efficiently. The 'challenging' behaviors are in fact requests for help, and these must be met and therapeutically answered by thoughtful, principled and respectful interventions, delivered through attuned and responsive touch. Be prepared to be changed forever in how you see a child's behavior, in what you think it means and how you can intervene directly with your own sensory and touch-based responses. As a parent, you will shift from attempts to stop and control behaviors to understanding, calming and using your relationship, presence and attunement to help your child suffer less, enjoy more and more fully grow. This will also change you in the same ways.

One of my core interests in the field of infant and early childhood mental health has been in professional and personal 'Formation' – how we grow in our understanding and capacity to promote growth and reduce suffering. In this Formation model, there are three interrelated domains in which we must grow – ways of 'KNOWING', ways of 'DOING' and ways of 'BEING WITH'. If you are guided by what you know (particularly when you fail to wonder about other ways of knowing), or if you simply deliver an intervention – "just do it" – without regard to *how* you are when intervening, you run the risk of ignoring elements of intervention (the 'relationship') that might be more important than the technique itself. This approach reflects a fundamental truth: when we engage in an intervention designed to promote growth and reduce suffering, what we KNOW (or think we know), influences what we DO (strategies, techniques, interventions), but these activities are delivered by another human being – another subject – so that HOW we are with the other – our affect, gestures, voice, posture, pacing, movement, TOUCH – are all the *media* of intervention. No person can attend to what they are doing without recognizing the impact of HOW they are doing what they are doing! There is unity of practice: knowing, doing and being with are inextricably linked (Costa, 2021).

Can you imagine a 'loving' touch that is only restricted to the tactile experience and not the affect and intent of the other? Can you separate a sensory intervention from *who* is delivering it and *how* it is delivered? Qigong Sensory Treatment (QST) reflects this unity of practice – an integration of intervention with the emotional experience of a relationship. Sensory touch is always relational and is never disembodied! It is two subjects interacting, sensing, relating, adapting and caring. When QST teaches the techniques of 'patting' and 'pressing', it gives parents a means by which to initiate a 'tactile conversation' with a child whose nervous system is immature or otherwise sensitive. But while you will learn the 12 core sensory/touch movements, it is critical not to consider these as intervention you can 'just do'. When a parent follows the protocol with sensitivity and attunement and engages in thoughtful and intentional touch patterns, what happens is the activation not just of touch receptors but of feeling states as well.

Many children with sensitive nervous systems develop (mal)adaptive patterns of behavior in attempting to reduce their stress levels. These patterns are often not effective because the child may require touch from another to organize their own sensory system. Donald Winnicott, the famed pediatrician turned psychoanalyst and infant mental health specialist, remarked that the "baby's first mirror is the mother's face!" Similarly, the parent can become the organizing 'other' for their child! Infants and young children who arrive in the world with disorganized nervous systems often cannot 'self-correct'. They need the sensitive, attuned and understanding guidance from another. Those others need a guide on what to know, what to do and how to 'be with' these children. QST provides that guide. Like the Winicottian 'mirror', the parent can become the relationship through which the child comes to know and enjoy themself sometimes for the first time.

A word about the power of 'pause'. Haven't we all wished that life had a pause button – a device that we could employ when events are unfolding too quickly, or when we are feeling that our and our children's stress levels are escalating at an overwhelming speed? Since we cannot change the operation of time, what we can do is, for the moment, disengage from being led by the events and instead make an intentional effort to slow down, look carefully and engage in 'wondering' about what is happening. Some, but not many, parents may have been helped by 'counting to 10' when they feel themselves losing it! And when you reach 10, what comes next? QST not only encourages the parent to pause or slow down; it offers very clear insights about what might be happening inside of themselves and how to respond in order to restore their own inner balance. Just as importantly, it gives parents insights and guidance to help restore balance in their child's inner experience of themselves. Through the understanding of neural pathways, the right blend of the parent's connection (relationship) and with the restorative sensory input (the 12 movements), QST will lead the child and parent to less stress and more mutual enjoyment. This begins with the knowledge of QST, the practice of 'pausing and wondering' in the moment, guided by the roadmap and the harnessing of an attuned relationship and sensitive, co-regulating touch.

Our world is buffeted by stress, and stress finds its way into our bodies, minds and spirits. When our ambient levels of stress encounter disorganized nervous systems – our own and our child's, we need to return to the 'containers' we have – our bodies. QST is rooted in a return to the body and in touch, our first and largest portal and our bridge to the world around us. Difficulties in sleep, appetite, digestion, regulation, orientation and attention, engagement and the capacity to be soothed and self-soothe – what Dr. Silva terms the "Early Self-Regulation Milestones" – turn our focus to the body and the ways in which our sensory systems function. The sensory language taught in QST reminds us that we come to help ourselves and others by attending to our sensory systems, and through connection, come to regulate, engage and communicate.

This book prepares the reader for a deep, reflective journey. Strap yourself into your seat for the ride of your life! You will learn about the theoretical foundations of QST, the domains of development in a child's life and the 12 core movements that comprise the touch guidelines. The section with 52 weekly letters anticipates the ups and downs that may be encountered and supports parents in effectively implementing QST over the course of a year. Parents are also given checklists and charts to measure progress over time.

QST is not a one-time intervention. It relies on an ongoing, consistent, predictable, attuned, sensitive, loving relationship between the child and another – often the parent, primary caregiver and other invested adults. Garofallou and Silva have remarkably written an easy-to-understand guide without ever losing the complexity of the subject. QST can be learned reliably and in a relatively short time, but it is not the speed of implementation but the consistency over time that leads to change. Many observed behavioral challenges have developed over time, and their underlying sensory difficulties have similarly existed for long periods. What has evolved over time will be helped over time. QST will reward the parent and practitioner for their dedication and patience.

The authors offer a wonderful metaphor. As you approach learning about QST, think of yourself as a "good gardener" rather than an "auto mechanic"! Your task is not to 'fix' your child, but to understand the nature of the problem and nurture the well-being of his or her sensory system from the bottom up – the soil in which we all are rooted.

I am grateful for this book and wish you good gardening!

Gerard Costa, PhD, DIR-C, IMH-E-Clinical®
Founding Director, Center for Autism and Early Childhood Mental Health
Professor, Department of Family Science and Human Development,
Montclair State University
President, Interdisciplinary Council on Development and Learning
January 2023

Bibliography

Costa, G. (2021). Reconceptualizing training as professional formation in the fields of autism and infant mental health. In N.L. Papaneophytou, & U.N. Das (Eds.), *Emerging Programs for Autism Spectrum Disorder*, Elsevier, Amsterdam, 211–236.

Shanker, S., & Barker, T. (2016). *Self-Reg: How to Help Your Child (and You) Break the Stress Cycle and Successfully Engage with Life*, Penguin Press, New York.

Preface and Acknowledgments

When Louisa and I began this book together, we both knew that she would not live to see its publication. Louisa had two fervent wishes for what she called this "time of completion" in her life. First was her joyous anticipation to meet her soon-to-be-born grandson. Next was her wish to extend, with this book, the lessons learned from her life's work with families and children with autism to the population of children she lovingly called "sensory kids". I feel blessed to have had the training and mentorship I received from Louisa and especially blessed for the months that we worked closely together on this book. Louisa's life was passionately dedicated to improving the health, development and lives of children and their families. Her legacy will live on in her unique understanding and treatment of children with developmental disorders. This book brings that wealth of knowledge, experience and perspective to a new group of children with a wide range of sensory and self-regulation difficulties.

Louisa asked that I extend her profound respect and gratitude to QST Master Trainers Sue Clayton and Linda Poling. She said that, clinically, she learned the most about sensory kids from Sue and Linda. I am forever grateful for Louisa's introduction to Sue, who proofed the text when Louisa no longer could. And, luckily for me, in the process, Sue became a respected colleague and dear friend across the miles between New Jersey and Australia. Louisa and I both extend our deepest gratitude to the families and children we have worked with over the years and all that they have taught us. I'm especially grateful to the group of families who participated as 'parent readers' at each step of this book. My goal was to always keep the book written in accessible, parent-friendly language, and their suggestions and comments were a guiding star to that end. I also want to thank QST Master Trainer Matt Elliott for his concise editing of the opening three chapters. Matt brought a unique set of skills to the task, including his work at Louisa's side during many of the QST research projects, his experience as a licensed acupuncturist and his past experience in early childhood special education and editing. He brought a unique clarity to those chapters. I also extend my appreciation to the group of QST Master Trainers who have shared their experience and expertise through contributions to the Weekly Letters found in Part III of this book.

In addition to Louisa, I've been blessed with several mentors in the early childhood mental health field whose wisdom, knowledge and expertise are suffused throughout the pages of this book. I was first introduced to the field by Dr. Gerard Costa over 20 years ago. He has continued to be a guiding light as a mentor, supervisor, colleague and now dear friend. His expertise, passion, compassion and dedication to the work of supporting families and children is monumental in our state, across the country and in the international community. My deepest gratitude to Gerry Costa and to Kathy Mulrooney for their wisdom, humanity and guidance in my work with mothers and their babies in residential drug rehabilitation. Together with the remarkable resilience I found in those mothers and babies, that experience taught me more about the power of touch in relationships, co-regulation and self-regulation than any book. I would also like to express my enduring appreciation to Drs. Stuart Shanker and Susan Hopkins at the MEHRIT Centre Self-Reg® initiative in Canada for continually deepening the understanding of self-regulation for all of us.

It is well-known that it 'takes a village to raise a child', but this also holds true for the village that has supported me during this book project. My gratitude and appreciation goes to Sophia Richman for introductions to Routledge and a very special thank you to Elaine Rollins for the generosity of her time, expertise and always-supportive guidance as my literary counsel. After all the years of knowing her as my sister-in-law, it was a lovely experience to see Elaine's impressive legal mind at work. Thank you to Brandon Hafer for his masterful graphics and always-timely help with the illustrations and graphics, and to Eileen McKeating for her generous help with infographics. A special thank-you goes to my editor at Routledge, Amanda Savage, for her steadfast patience with the many delays of the manuscript. I also extend my thanks to Katya Porter, my editorial assistant, for her instantaneous responses to any and all questions, even across a five-hour time difference. A similar thank-you goes to my friends and family for the patience shown when hearing all too infrequently from me during the lengthy process of writing. And my sincere thanks go to my colleagues at the Center for Autism and Early Childhood Mental Health at Montclair State University for their always-enthusiastic support. It is a gift to work with such a bright, impressive and tirelessly dedicated group of professionals.

I end with the deepest sense of gratitude and awe at the fierce dedication, patience and support of my beloved husband, Jim. His gift to me and the unfolding of this book is more enormous than I could have ever imagined. He challenged me at every turn to think more broadly and more deeply, and even when I resisted, he challenged me more. His beautifully disciplined mind and keen eye for the crafting of thought and poetic turn of words often captured the deeper complexities and meanings of this book and are responsible for its readable flow. His unending patience and uniquely honed expertise in editing made it possible for my thoughts and words to unfold through a process that made them better than what I could ever have accomplished alone. The process of writing and re-writing that passed between us was a gift beyond measure.

Louisa understood and trusted in 'the process' inherent in a project such as this more than anyone I've known, and the experience of working with Louisa, Jim and all those who have made contributions leave me with a deepened sense of gratitude and respect for each of them and that process. I extend my greetings and warmest wishes to each parent or professional who has this book in their hands. My hope is that you will find here an enriching process for you and your family or in your work with clients.

Linda Garofallou, December 2022

Welcome to QST!

This book empowers parents with an at-home, hands-on intervention to effectively address their children's sensory, self-regulation and related behavioral problems. It is focused on children who are under the age of six, however much of it can be applied to older children as well. With Louisa Silva's over 35 years of practicing medicine and Linda Garofallou's 20+ years working with families and children with developmental disorders, what stands out the most in our minds is the love, energy and resilience that parents bring to raising their children, especially when that includes the symptoms associated with sensory, behavioral and developmental challenges. What parents need most is clear, simple information about what they can do to help. You already have that trusted physician for your child and have probably consulted a variety of intervention specialists. Our book offers a new perspective on these difficulties and shows you what you can do at home to help. It is not a substitute for medical care or other clinical interventions; it is a complement to them.

A Different Approach

Most parents understand that just trying to 'manage' or 'control' difficult behaviors rarely works very well. We see these behaviors as stemming directly from sensory and self-regulation difficulties, not from what often gets mislabeled as 'bad behavior'. Qigong Sensory Treatment (QST) puts parents at the center of the intervention. Our approach gives you the skills to calm and organize your child's sensory experience, so she is better able to handle the ups and downs and stresses of the day without triggering those all-too-familiar behavioral storms. When you shift your perspective from controlling behaviors to calming and regulating the stress response cascading through your child's body that has triggered them, you free your child to develop the inner capacities to regulate her own body, emotions and behavior. And that is the doorway to renewed development on a healthier track. With this new perspective, you will come to not only see your child's behaviors differently you will see your child differently.

Children with sensory and behavioral issues represent a tremendously varied group with an equally wide range of symptoms and conditions, but we think you'll recognize your child's particular sensory picture as you read and learn how this book can help. Louisa's autism research has shown that sensory difficulties, no matter the cause, are best resolved at the periphery, in the skin, where the nervous system touches and interacts with the outside world. This vast set of nerves, just under the skin's surface, is the gateway from the outer world to inner sensory and brain organization. And a parent's natural caring touch is essential to activating that organization.

DOI: 10.4324/9781003360421-1

But an immature sensory nervous system often leaves a child in a hyper-reactive state, so that the very touch that is crucial for her development can feel overwhelming, irritating or even painful. It is as if your child is profoundly dehydrated but rejects the very water she needs to thrive. QST helps you minimize or eliminate those sensory discomforts so your child can take in what she desperately needs from you – your calming presence and organizing touch. The first step in minimizing those discomforts is to use your skilled touch, organized and delivered through the daily QST routine, which provides you with a kind of 'sensory language' to go directly to the root of the problems. That gives you the power to speak to your child in the language of touch – a 'sensory solution' to your child's sensory and self-regulation problems.

This book is dedicated to giving you that power, *in your own home*, to be an active participant in your child's therapeutic progress. We live in a culture that looks to specialists and experts to solve our problems. Like medical specialists who treat only one part of the body or another, each specialist treats only part of the problem. While they offer necessary and invaluable help, it is easy for parents to feel disempowered from believing what they know to be true and trusting that they hold the whole picture of their child. Our belief is that the best approach is a combination of the two: to consult the best experts, but to do so without falling into the trap of becoming disempowered or passive.

QST gives you the skills to normalize your child's sensory responses that help her find her way back to a calm, receptive state, a place where she is ready and eager to listen and learn. Once that happens, your touch becomes both therapy and reward, sensory issues and behavior improve and you have a tool to connect and help your child feel safe, calm and open to the world around her. And while all of this is happening, something even bigger is taking place – the building and strengthening of your child's connection to and relationship with you.

So, What is QST?

Qigong Sensory Treatment is an at-home program designed especially for parents that incorporates everything we have learned to help you integrate and regulate your child's sensory and behavioral difficulties by:

> using your *attuned* responsiveness . . .
> through your caring, skilled touch . . .
> that travels along the special C-tactile highway . . .
> directly from *you* to your child's brain . . .
> to help regulate sensory triggers . . .
> so your child can achieve a relax-and-relate mode, which over time . . .
> leads to a better capacity for self-regulation and greater sensory maturity.

The treatment integrates approaches to sensory problems from both modern Western and Traditional Chinese Medicine. "Q" is the Chinese medicine part – it stands for Qigong, pronounced "chee-gong". It is an ancient form of Chinese medical healing that includes massage and movement used to improve health, energy and circulation. "ST" stands for Sensory Treatment. QST is a treatment for the sensory problems that can stand in the way of your child's healthy development.

QST was created by Louisa Silva, a practicing physician who was trained in both Western and Chinese medicine. What made her unique is that she was also a researcher who conducted university-based scientific studies steeped in a holistic view of a child's development. Her QST autism research protocols have been validated in the Western tradition by extensive research, the latest of which is a three-year US Department of Health and Human Services – Maternal Child Health Bureau (www.QSTI.org/published-studies/) research study (2016). Blending an integrated mix of East and West, she created a protocol supported by current research and based on a system that has stood the test of centuries. The distinctive contribution that Louisa brought from the Oriental medicine perspective is that a parent's skilled touch could establish a form of sensory communication and an 'organized connection' between their child's brain and the world around them.

   We are excited to be able to make this program available to everyone. When we first began this work in Oregon, we were only able to help families in our geographic area. Now, we can offer it to you wherever you live. QST books have been translated into six languages and are used throughout the world. We wish you the best success! If you have problems or questions, contact information is available in Appendix D – Getting Personalized Help. Write us, email us or check our website (www.QSTI.org/). We want to help you and your child unlock his or her potential and join in all that the world has to offer.

Linda Garofallou – Montclair, New Jersey
Dr. Louisa Silva – Salem, Oregon [Deceased]

What's in This Book?

We know that parents get the bests results when they have:

- a good background and understanding of sensory problems;
- a confidence in their touch technique and the resources to address troubleshooting difficulties that can arise; and
- week-by-week support with short, easy-to-digest guidance that reinforces their progress.

Our goal is to provide all three. To do that, we've divided this book into three sections. **Part I** pulls back the curtain on sensory problems by giving you a fuller understanding of what's going on inside your child and of the role that touch, natural development and especially **you** can play in making it better. **Part II** gives you everything you need to learn the QST method at home and provides a host of practical tips and helpful guides to meet those everyday difficult situations. Finally, **Part III** is designed to stay right there with you, week by week, offering timely weekly letters to guide you through your first year of QST and ensure that you get the most benefits. We've included a comprehensive index that can serve as a reference for addressing specific questions at any time. And, to help measure your progress over time, you will find simple checklists and a do-it-yourself progress chart to easily record and follow your child's growth and progress throughout the year.

Part I – Pulling Back the Curtain

This first part is designed to help you understand the roots of your child's sensory and behavioral problems, learn how you can help and feel more secure and effective as you begin the QST hands-on routine.

Chapter 1 gives you a road map to understand how your child's sensory and self-regulation problems are directly linked to related behavioral problems. You'll see that what appears to be challenging behavior is often the result of an immature sensory nervous system that leaves your child easily overwhelmed. We take a closer look at your child's sensory triggers and how they cause over-reactivity and an automatic flight into a stress 'survival mode'. You'll see that when she is in that state, she is not just 'behaving badly' or pushing you away – she is essentially pushing away the stimulation that is over-loading her nervous system. Finally, we look at the importance of helping your child find her way back to feeling safe, calm and receptive to you – that place where all connection and learning takes place.

Chapter 2 focuses on self-regulation and its connection to sensory problems. We explain what self-regulation is and why it is so important for every child, but especially for the sensory child. Louisa's research has studied this critical area and she has outlined four basic developmental steps, the "Early Self-Regulation Milestones", essential achievements for every child in the first three years of life. You'll see how your child's sensory problems can interfere with reaching these essential milestones and how that can lead to problems with emotions and behavior that can cascade into social and learning problems. Most importantly, you'll learn how the QST technique can help your child reclaim those capacities for self-regulation that will put her on the path to healthier development.

In **Chapter 3**, we look at the critical importance of a parent's touch for their child's healthy development. We start by looking at how our culture has in many ways lost an understanding of just how important and effective a parent's touch can be for improving an immature sensory system. We take a look at some of the newest findings from neuroscience to see how touch, of all the senses, provides a unique and direct pathway to the key parts of the brain that play a central role in sensory organization.

Chapter 4 is for those parents who are interested in knowing what QST does and how it works. It takes a deeper look at how Louisa's unique perspective brought a radical new way of thinking about sensory problems, one that focuses on parent touch to effect sensory growth and strengthen inner capacities for self-regulation. You will see how the patting and pressing movements used in QST create the basis of a non-verbal touch language that you can use to communicate with your child in a way that goes deeper than words. With that language you can 'speak and listen to' your child in the sensory-feeling language that she best understands.

Chapter 5 extends the idea of a sensory language to include that wide range of choices and responses you make, both during QST and in everyday interactions as well. You'll see the all-important goal of your child's growing capacity for self-regulation through a new lens – as a balance between attuned connection and safe boundaries. Your growing ability to adjust between these two critical elements is powerfully communicated to your child. As your awareness of your child's sensory language grows, so does your awareness of new, intentional and effective responses to provide that balance. We tell the story of how two different parents work to find this balance, how that impacts their child and how you can re-set that balance for your child to help them return to a path of growing self-regulation.

Chapter 6 is all about you and how you can foster your own self-regulation to bring the best version of yourself to QST. We'll help you focus on the kinds of simple questions to ask yourself and what you can do to keep your own inner balance, and how that balance will allow you to stay sensitively connected to your child's cues, while maintaining good boundaries and staying in the moment with your child. You'll see that *who* you are as you do the treatment creates a direct link, through what neuroscientists call the 'interbrain', between you and your child. It is a link that conveys your own success at maintaining inner balance directly into her growing capacity to self-regulate.

Part II – Learning QST at Home

Chapters 7 and 8 help you learn the QST daily routine – how to get started (**Chapter 7**) and how to do the routine (**Chapter 8**). We've included detailed, step-by-step instructions and diagrams showing how to do each of the 12 movements that comprise the daily routine along with an understanding of the purpose and intention behind each step. Links to online videos clearly demonstrate how each step is done.

Chapters 9 through 11 are about putting it all together and learning the sensory method in greater detail. You'll learn to read your child's body and behavioral cues (**Chapter 9**) and learn how to adapt your touch technique to enhance your effectiveness. We include chapters on how to work through the difficult spots (**Chapter 10**), developing skills and sensory solutions for challenging behaviors (**Chapter 11**) as well as some extra techniques to help your child get through the day. Together, these three chapters present important skills and tools that will help you feel reassured when faced with the natural uncertainties about whether you are doing things correctly. Our goal is to give you all that you need to feel confident and stick with the daily routine so you can see and feel the benefits for you and your child. To help you along the way, we've also included some handy tools to help with your child's most challenging behaviors.

Chapter 12 looks at those essential building blocks of healthy development that we may overlook in our busy day-to-day lives – diet, sleep and rhythmic daily routines. These are the easily forgotten parts of the day that, when absent, can serve as hidden triggers that contribute to your child's behavioral symptoms. You'll see how, with a few simple improvements in diet and nutrition and the creation of rhythm and structure in your day-to-day activities, you can provide an atmosphere of order and safety in daily life while identifying and removing any agitating triggers.

Part III – Guiding Your Way With 52 Weekly Letters

In this final section, we walk with you through the first year of QST by providing short weekly letters that are timed to address key issues that we've seen many parents experience along the way. The letters are written to take just minutes of your time each week. There are also letters from parents who offer their helpful experiences as well as advice and from QST Master Trainers who offer their years of expertise. The letters cover topics such as mastering the basics, maintaining daily regulation, staying consistent, marking progress, extra techniques for difficult behavior, QST for children with specific medical needs and a year-end round up. There are simple charts and checklists to easily measure your progress over the year.

Finally, the **Appendices** at the back of the book provide a wide range of tools, resources and useful information. There you will find the *QST Sensory Movement Chart*, a *Troubleshooting Guide* and *Access to Online Instructional Videos and Support Materials*, along with information about where to find personalized QST help. Also included is a 'how-to' guide to finding or creating a local support group and a template for how QST can be integrated as a valuable asset into early intervention programs. Next, an appendix highlights the key results from Louisa's QST autism research as it applies to children with sensory and behavioral difficulties. The final appendix contains a link to access the online instructional videos and support materials for the book.

Thoughts Before You Begin

For Parents

We have put a lot of information into this book to make it a complete resource. But just as every child has their own unique set of sensory problems and resulting behaviors, every parent has a unique way that helps them to best learn something new. So, we've written our book in three sections so you can choose the way to learn that works best for you.

We highly recommend that every parent read the first six chapters in Part I – Pulling Back the Curtain because each chapter gives you, step-by-step, a deeper picture of what sits at the root of your child's difficult behaviors and will change the way you 'see' your child. These chapters give you valuable insights about how QST, in your hands, opens new, more organized and integrated pathways of regulation for your child so you can see 'behind' the behaviors and 'beyond' any diagnosis that your child has been given. You'll find that seeing your child through this new lens gives you one of the most important keys to your success, your own intentions and your skilled observations.

But people learn differently, and if you are a parent who just needs to jump in and get started, you can go directly to Part II – Learning QST at Home. Use the diagrams, instructions and Louisa's online step-by-step video lessons to begin to learn and implement the daily routine with your child. If you jump ahead, we still encourage you to come back to those chapters in Part I because QST is much more than just *what* you do. You don't even have to read this book from beginning to end. QST is not something that you learn all at once. You can go step-by-step in the way that suits you best and put it all together over time. Everything new has a natural learning curve and it's easy to feel overwhelmed in the beginning. But trust us – it gets easier! Actually, QST is surprisingly simple and very effective when it's done in a consistent and intentional way.

This book is designed as a compliment to medical and clinical interventions, not a substitute for them. It is written for a broad range of children with sensory and behavioral difficulties. If you have any question or have a child with a medical condition, please consult with your physician before beginning QST [see Appendix C – Contraindications to QST Sensory Protocol, page 210].

Thoughts Before You Begin

For Clinicians and Professionals

Written primarily for parents, this book is also designed as a comprehensive text and reference for clinicians and professionals who work with families and children with sensory and self-regulation problems and their behavioral manifestations. Conceived and designed as a daily, at-home, parent-delivered intervention, our research model trains and certifies professionals (QST Trainers) in the hands-on method to work with the parent-child dyad. The role of the trained and certified clinician is to help the parent learn to tailor their own at-home touch technique to their child's individual sensory and regulatory needs, most often required in the early months of treatment. Professionals who may benefit from this book include those pursuing certification in the QST method, as well as any clinician interested in learning more about the technique itself, or who wants a deeper understanding of sensory and regulatory dysfunctions and their related behavioral problems.

Our theoretical focus, often overlooked in today's literature, is that these sensory dysregulations are remediated through what we term a 'sensory language'. We focus on a special form of tactile communication through which parents transmit to the child, in ways that will be elaborated further in this book, the underlying building blocks of self-regulation. We are convinced that children's sensory problems require a sensory solution, and we start our intervention at the developmental foundation of that hierarchical pyramid of sensory modalities: touch.

Theory. Our approach sits on four interrelated pillars: touch, affective neuropathways, energy flow as understood through Traditional Chinese Medicine and the critical importance of the parent-child relationship. We see 'parent touch' as the first pillar, providing a direct physiologic and affective pathway to key regulatory areas of the child's brain and neurological organization. That is, we see skilled parent touch as the key intervention that, when properly structured and attuned to a child's body and behavioral cues, completes the circuit from brain to behavior. Touch travels through critical neuropathways to the brain, creates energetic patterns of organization and structure and, when transmitted through the relationship, carries the essential messages that underpin co-regulation. Touch sits at the center of our theory (and practice), and the normalization of that touch is the key to our therapeutic intervention.

The primacy of touch leads us to our second pillar, the recently discovered C-tactile afferents that provide an 'affective neuropathway' that travels directly to and impacts the neuro-biological roots of sensory difficulties. To date, the understanding of touch has been limited to its discriminatory functions – providing our tactile perception of the world, informing our sensorimotor functions, creating a detailed body map and orchestrating the other senses. The discovery of C-tactile fibers adds an affective, feeling-based element to that touch signal, providing emotional and interpersonal depth to sensory input. Now imparted with affective meaning, that tactile experience broadens the capacities of the basic body map, creating a relational guide by which the child can both integrate the sensory array and build an experienced feeling of a 'self' that has its own identity. That added dimension gives the capacity for a 'felt' emotional experience of touch that would otherwise be mere sensory data.

To better conceptualize the nature of that structure and how it can be organized, we employ a therapeutic model based on Chinese medicine. That leads us to the third pillar in our theory, 'energy flow'. In Chinese medicine, this is understood as 'qi'. From the Western perspective, it is simply energy. The model of the flow of this energy provides parents and clinicians with a way to conceptualize and implement a dynamic intervention where the technique can rapidly shift to address the changing needs of both the child's sensory nervous system and the felt interpersonal relationship. We see the underlying sensory organizational problem and its regulatory and neurological components through this lens of facilitating energy flow. As you will see, two outwardly simple touch techniques, patting and pressing, can be combined to enhance and open blocks in this energy flow that establish the foundations of a sensory organization that meets the child's regulatory needs in the moment. And because touch is a reciprocal experience, it embeds the relationship right into the intervention.

Which brings us to the fourth pillar – the critical element of our theoretical approach – the parent-child 'relationship' itself. Since the sensory organization that QST imparts is first conveyed through informed and structured touch, the knowledge, intention, feeling and sensitive source of that knowledge and intention is first consolidated in the parent and then conveyed through the relationship. A great deal of this book is focused on the caregiver because it is the parent or clinician who must first be centered, organized and attuned. Once established, that structure is imparted directly to the child.

We believe that these four pillars – touch, affective neuropathways, energy flow and the primacy of the parent-child relationship – also offer the clinician a broader basis on which to assess behavioral problems associated with sensory difficulties. Typical diagnoses attributed to 'sensory' children very often lead parents (and clinicians) to focus on behaviors and symptoms, yet do not adequately consider the sensory, regulatory and developmental needs that sit at the heart of those conditions. Once officially diagnosed, the child can identify with and 'become' that label, while the clinician's perceived options for conceptualizing the case and choice of treatment modality can likewise become limited and exclusionary. We feel that our model helps to open the clinician's range of thinking, offering an expanded array of choices and a more fluid-dynamic approach to making interventions.

Clinical method. Tactile communication with a child is conceived as a sensory 'conversation' in which there is an ever evolving and increasingly synchronized back-and-forth, non-verbal flow through which co-regulation is transmitted. A good conversation of this type is comprised of quickly alternating affective and tactile 'calls and responses' and, as with any good interaction, each partner has the option to lead, follow or re-direct. The child leads by indicating through her reactions to touch, mood and movements which type of touch creates greater or lesser sensory overload. She follows when the appropriate touch technique enables her nervous system to fall into a state of receptive calm, and she re-directs when she signals, either by action or affect, what she needs in the moment to sustain that calm. The parent or clinician leads by providing the intention to normalize touch through a structured protocol. They follow by adeptly adapting to the child's signals of overload. And they re-direct by rapidly altering course to establish more tolerable and accessible forms of touch.

We feel that this model helps to resolve a fundamental paradox of a touch-based treatment – that the treatment can re-trigger the very problems with touch that it was designed to ameliorate. The answer is to be found in the skilled clinician's or parent's ability to quickly shift away from tactile overload – *but not away from touch itself.* Such attuned shifts convey to the child that her painful or sensitive reactions will be respected in two ways – the adult will retreat from overload in response to the child's cues yet will continue the contact by intervening with a calming tactile alternative. In this way, sensitivity to touch is slowly normalized, first by being respected as legitimate and then being offered and replaced with an ameliorative affective tactile connection. It is through tactile conversations such as these that co-regulation and ultimately the capacity for self-regulation is transmitted.

The model makes room for the certified clinician to sensitively press forward when a child protests yet remains open to immediately changing the touch technique as body and behavioral cues signal sensory nervous system overload. To achieve this, the parent and/or clinician consistently monitors to avoid sending the child into survival mode, remaining fully connected while not avoiding difficult areas of sensitivity that elicit protest. The message conveyed to the overwhelmed child is that she is understood, supported and respected while, at the same time, offered a better sensory avenue toward connection. It is the adult who embodies and resolves the paradox of a touch-based treatment when they simultaneously respect the child's discomfort yet persist toward a better touch alternative. In that moment, the child's experience of touch is normalized with affection and connection and thereby re-claimed. It is touch's affective reciprocity, reflexivity and sensitivity that sets the stage for this commonplace, yet remarkable achievement.

For Professional Certification in the QST Method

If you are a clinician or a professional who would like to be trained and certified in the QST method, please see the Qigong Sensory Training Institute website for information and qualifications required for the QSTI certification course (www.qsti.org/professional-training-and-certification/). The certification course is based on the theory and practice of the research-based QST Autism Protocol, including a four-week course of theory and practice, followed by five months of clinical case supervision with a family who has a child diagnosed with autism. Also, please refer to your state licensing board for any specific requirements that you must meet to provide professional hands-on treatment. This book is not intended to replace the QST Trainer certification and cannot be used by clinicians in practice without prior certification by QSTI.

Part I

Pulling Back the Curtain

Chapter 1

Behavior Through a Sensory Lens

Do you remember going to the amusement park fun house as a child? The floors look slanted one way, but take a step and gravity pulls you the opposite way. Your image and everything around you are distorted. Lights flash, sounds are jarring and things jump out at you without notice. All of your senses are bombarded with intense, confusing information. But you adjust and in time it can all feel exciting and invigorating.

Now think about that fun house again, but this time say you've had a frustrating day at work, a bad night's sleep, your nerves are on edge and you are at the end of your rope. Just think about how different your experience would be. Certainly not excited and invigorated! You need it to stop. You'd be quick to over-react, overwhelmed and exhausted by each new assault on your senses. What was fun before is now threatening. You would want out and no one could stand in your way, even if you had to fight!

You've just had a picture of what sensory overload is like for your child. For you, a good night's sleep will re-set your nervous system. But it won't re-set his. Why? Because at their root, sensory and related self-regulation and behavioral problems often stem from an immature sensory nervous system that leaves children with senses that are easily stressed. Once this happens, their brains switch out of calm-listening mode and into a sensory stress mode that can rapidly move to sensory overload where children get hyper, cry, lash out or shut down. Most importantly, they've stopped listening and being receptive to you because *their thinking-problem-solving mind has turned off.* When sensory overload is at its most extreme, you can see prolonged behavioral meltdowns along with either extreme sensitivity or total withdrawal. When those meltdowns or tantrums occur, a parent's natural instinct is to try to control the behavior.

But that leads to a parent's dilemma. Your natural attempts to soothe through touch or words can result in the exact opposite of what you intended, triggering even more over-stimulation and meltdowns that can go on for hours. If you try to exert control to fix the problem, it just makes the problem worse. That's because the root of the problem is *not his behavior* but his developmentally immature nervous system that cannot tolerate even normal sensory input. Sensory problems are *not a choice* your child is making, and the behaviors they lead to are not choices either. Those behaviors are deeply ingrained, automatic survival reactions. If he could tell you in words he would, but his behavior *is* his language! Our job is to help you learn that language.

Through an understanding of his cues and with this survival mode lens, you will see that what looked like intentional behavior is really a kind of automatic threat response that needs to be

DOI: 10.4324/9781003360421-3

calmed before your child can get back on a healthy track. This is a crucial point for parents to understand. When in this state, your child is *not misbehaving or being willful*. He is reacting to the confusion, helplessness and overwhelming feelings of sensory overload. Once you see this difference, you are free to deal with the *real* problem by addressing your child's underlying need – to reduce what is causing the sensory stressors and create a sense of safety, both in yourself and your child. That is at the heart of making a lasting change.

While this book will often zero in on the most extreme behaviors because they can be the most difficult to deal with, our real focus is to give you the skills to help strengthen and mature your child's senses and nervous system responses, to help him be more resilient to sensory stimulation and more open to what he needs most in times of stress: your support to feel safe. You picked up this book to learn a skill to help your child with sensory, emotional and related behavioral problems and to find ways to respond effectively when your child is stressed or reactive. With QST, you will learn body-based techniques that not only help regulate difficult sensory behaviors, but also address the underlying causes. Together, they will quiet the moment by bringing a sense of security and calm and, more importantly, will organize the senses over time to help resolve future episodes.

Reframing behavior shifts the focus to looking at the reasons behind the cause of that behavior. See a child differently and you see a different child.

Dr. Stuart Shanker (2016)

An Immature Sensory System

Let's begin with how your child's sensory nervous system matures under ideal conditions. In the womb, we develop the eight basic senses: touch, vision, sound, taste and smell plus the two senses that give us an awareness about where our body is in space (proprioception) and our sense of movement (kinesthetics), along with the sense that helps us feel what is going on inside our body (interoception). All of these senses are directly linked through the autonomic nervous system, the part of the nervous system that controls involuntary processes in our body and responds to threats.

At birth, healthy newborns have a highly active sensory system that triggers alarm bells at slight changes in temperature, pressure or hunger. When a sensory alarm goes off, the baby cries. Parents are hard-wired to recognize this distress, remove the problem and soothe their baby. As this back and forth recurs many times each day, parent and newborn come to know each other. The baby comes to experience that whatever the stress, his parent will help him get back to feeling comfortable, safe and calm. Most importantly, through this process of parent-regulation, the baby's nervous system 'learns' more mature responses to regulate itself so the alarm bells are triggered less and less frequently. With repeated positive co-regulating experiences, the nervous system grows stronger and more capable of tolerating sensory input without getting overwhelmed. By the time the child reaches preschool, his sensory system is ready to deal with the new experiences of school and learning without excess reactivity.

But children with immature sensory systems remain reactive and prone to significant overwhelm. Even with a parent's most caring efforts, children respond to sensory stress more like an infant or a much younger child. There can be many causes for this immaturity, including genetics, early experience of injury, trauma, environmental exposure or prolonged stress. Most often, there are multiple simultaneous causes that interact and prevent a child's nervous system from maturing in this normative way. Whatever the cause, it leaves children unable to develop a healthy resilience to stimulation, leading, in extreme cases, to tantrums or meltdowns, even in what may appear to us as a normal environment. Because each child's nervous system is unique, each will have a different emotional and behavioral response to sensory overload. For some who are over-reactive, alarm bells get triggered too quickly and strongly. For the under-reactive, alarm bells get triggered when sensory input is not registered or processed well. Coming to understand your child's particular triggers will help you to better guide your child to a state of calm and self-regulation.

When our son would go into one of his meltdowns when we were out and about, we had learned to take him home. It was just not worth it trying to soldier through. Over time, we've figured out some of his main triggers – new places, family gatherings, certain noises like the buzzing of fluorescent lights, certain clothing, and we'd try to stay clear of those things to prevent the meltdowns. Now with QST we can go out without all of the tantrums and hours long meltdowns.

Mother of a 3-year-old

Fast and Slow Sensory Triggers

Most children experiencing immature sensory responses have alarm bells that are triggered too quickly and easily. It is as if a slight tap on the gas pedal makes them go from 0–100 mph in one second. Before you even know what has happened, your child can lash out or have a meltdown. Often, this behavior may look more like that of a much younger child. In fact, the hallmark of a dysregulated trigger is that it fires at an age or in situations where that shouldn't normally be a problem. For example, the sound of a door slamming may upset an infant but it shouldn't upset an 8-year-old. The excitement of a birthday party should not cause undue emotional distress or agitation for a 6-year-old. Your child's triggers may also become more sensitive when he is tired and his energy reserves are low, which can result in changes in his sensitivity from day to day or even hour to hour. As you are reading this, your child's own personal sensory triggers are probably already coming to mind – noises that are too loud, lights that are too bright or the wrong kind of touch on a particular body area, like ears, fingers or toes.

For children who are over-reactive, these seemingly ordinary sensations of sound and touch feel more intense and, more importantly, can signal threat or danger, even when they come from the most caring parent. These children are often referred to as hyper- or over-reactive and may even be labeled as 'over-sensitive' or 'picky'. By preschool, their over-reactivity to stimuli can leave them feeling anxious, irritable, angry or fearful. This can result in reactions as mild as flushing of the cheeks, wobbly legs and butterflies in the stomach. Or it might lead all the way to shutting down, biting, kicking, hitting or prolonged temper tantrums.

While most kids with immature nervous systems fall into the over-reactive category with fast triggers, some actually have 'slow' triggers. These are children with hypo- or under-reactive nervous systems. It can take them two minutes to respond to that same press of the gas pedal before their sensory systems even register and, while it may not look like it, this lag can also cause inner stress. That's because children sense the mismatch when they are not responding in the same ways as the people around them. They need a great deal of sensory input, often in the form of more intense physical activity, to help them feel or register the same level of input to their brains. You may see them as being passive, disinterested or unaffected, but what they really need is a lot more of the right kind of sensory input to get their systems going. These are children who love being tossed in the air over and over, or love to jump on furniture or on bouncy balls. This need for greater stimulation can be confusing to parents because their child's behavior can also appear to be hyper-sensitive and hyper-reactive to stimuli when, in fact, they are really under-sensitive. Such children are not overwhelmed, they actually are *seeking out* the sensory input that they crave in order to get their system working and to relieve the tension.

Whether too fast or too slow, if left without intervention, the repeating patterns of overwhelm and reactivity caused by those triggers can, over time, lay down brain circuit pathways and patterns for interactions that start to define how your child relates to others and even defines how he sees himself. So, it's important to recognize your child's own personal triggers because the first step in any positive intervention is to identify the source of those triggers and to remove him from that environment. As you continue to minimize these stimuli you will be taking an important step in breaking the cycle of chronically re-stressing his system. Over time and with your positive interventions, his sensory system will mature, and he will likely be able to return to those situations without being re-triggered.

Survival Mode

Our primary concern is aggression, which we have seen in our child since age two. He is a very bright, sensitive, highly imaginative child who also struggles with frequent overwhelm and anger, based at least in part, on sensory issues. He has a very difficult time regulating when he is triggered and some of the triggers we know of include clothing irritations and distressing sounds (baby brother crying, dog barking). He can go from '0–100' quickly and appears to shut-down at times, making it difficult or impossible to communicate with him in those moments.

Mother of a 5-year-old

This mother's story will sound very familiar to many parents. It shows how quickly sensory problems can move from simple sensory stress to complete overload resulting in the full 'fight-flight-or-freeze' survival response. Many people believe that this survival mode is our first natural response to threat. It is not. A child's *very first* response when faced with sensory stress or threat, is to turn to their parent for safety and comfort. Ideally, that turns off the survival response. But for children who have *rapid triggers* and entrenched survival-mode patterns, even the most caring and responsive parent's attention might not reach them before they escalate and lash out or push away the support they desperately need. Our neurobiological survival mechanisms function many times faster than our conscious brains. Sensory triggers fire before we can do anything about them and can preclude support by even the most attentive parent. On the other hand, *slow triggers* leave them under-responsive and unavailable to even the most patient and loving parents. In both cases, an automatic defensive mode sets in and the overwhelming sense of threat gets automatically channeled into a survival reaction – fight, flight or freeze. Fight means that we lash out to protect ourselves. Flight means we run away or try to avoid the situation. But when neither of these two works, a child can literally freeze in place. For kids, that often means shutting down completely.

When a child is in fight, flight or freeze mode, a cascade of stress hormones floods the body. This response is hard-wired in his brain and his behavior is totally on auto-pilot. Once this stress response starts, these hormones can stay in the blood stream for longer periods of time than for typically-developing children. That makes it difficult or impossible for them to stop problem behaviors which can then go on and on until those stress hormones wash out of their system. When a child with intense and sensitive triggers repeatedly gets stuck in a state driven by stress neuro-hormones, it can have compounding effects on an already immature nervous system.

We're sure you've had the experience this mother described when she said it is "impossible to communicate with him" during those times. That's because when a child is in the fight-flight-or-freeze mode he is operating automatically out of his survival brain. He can't take advantage of your presence or your efforts to help him regulate and feel safe. His 'thinking-connecting-relating brain' has shut down, along with his capacity to hear what you are saying. And that 'shut-down' is quite literally true because when a child is in survival mode, the muscles in his inner ear actually constrict and are tuned more to low range sounds of threat, not to the range of your normal spoken voice. He may look like he is hearing you at those times, but he is not. If you raise your voice in frustration, make demands or show anger, *he only hears your tone* as a threat and that deepens the automatic stress reaction he is locked in at that moment (Porges & Furman, 2011). Only when he is calm do the inner ear muscles finally relax so he can hear your spoken voice again. Knowing that can free you from pressing him to listen and allow you to be more attuned to helping him get back to a state where he is *capable* of listening.

In doing Self-Reg we learn to look at others and ourselves with 'soft eyes'. As we learn to read the signs of stress behavior, the soft eyes just come.

Dr. Susan Hopkins (2016)

Each child has different sensory triggers and differing levels of reactivity, so not all fight-flight-or-freeze reactions are always extreme. For example, when a child has mild over-reactivity to touch and muscle sensations, a stress response might show up as a tummy ache or a cold clammy feeling. For a child with a moderate level of reactivity to certain sounds, a flight reaction may show up as withdrawal in class or difficulty paying attention to his teacher. What's important when it comes to fight, flight or freeze reactions is not how extreme the behavior is but recognizing what's happening *inside* your child that's causing these problems in the first place. Once we understand that, we can begin to help him get out of survival mode, whether it's intense or mild.

Which Mode Is Your Child's Brain In?

Knowing which mode your child is in will help you to understand what your child is reacting to and what he needs from you to reach that state of calm, open receptivity. You can often tell which stress mode your child is in by just looking at his body language, facial expression and behavior. Table 1.1 below helps with what to look for. Notice that when your child is in his comfort zone (relax-and-relate), he will appear receptive to you and the people around him: he looks directly in your eyes, his body is relaxed, he makes eye contact and his face is content. These body signals

Table 1.1 Which mode is your child's brain in?

	Relax-and-Relate	**Fight**	**Flight**	**Freeze**
Body Language	Your child is relaxed and engaged with what is happening around him	Defensive posture Hitting, pinching, kicking, biting, spitting	Shrinking posture Hiding behavior Running away	Standing off to the side and staring Sitting and 'planting' in one spot
Facial Expression	Engaged Making eye contact and listening Healthy skin tone	Angry	Scared Pale skin tone	Blank expression

show that his brain and thinking processes are open, engaged and ready to learn. He is relatively free of sensory stress. But, when in the high stress zone (fight-flight-or-freeze), your child can't cope.

Comfort Zone or High Stress Zone

These three modes of behavior, fueled by the stress hormones flooding his body, are pretty easy to see in their extremes; hitting, running away or freezing in place are the most obvious examples. Willfulness, rejection and aggression are all also forms of fight-flight behavior. With more moderate sensitivity, you may see irritability, shyness or withdrawal. There are many shades of survival mode and some of them can be quite subtle. For example, a freeze response may at first seem like a state of calm but if you look more closely, you will see a blank expression on your child's face, staring off into space and a lack of responsivity.

There is another, recently identified stress mode that can also be hard to recognize. Outwardly, it looks like a state of calm, but it masks a major stress response happening inside. It's called 'appease' mode. Here, a child appears to be cooperating in a positive and compliant way but is only acting this way to placate and avoid conflict. Inwardly, he is overwhelmed and stress hormones are flooding his body. Any of these stress modes can be deceptive to a concerned parent. So, you can see why it is important to learn your child's unique way of expressing his feelings through his body cues. In fact, your attunement to non-verbal body language is such an important part of QST that we have devoted an entire chapter to it. Chapter 9 provides you with a comprehensive list of the important body and behavioral cues to watch for and what to do when you see them.

Relax-and-Relate Mode

Fortunately, there is another system built into the brain that keeps us from being locked in survival mode when we feel threatened or unsafe. We all have this special and highly evolved way to defend against stress. It is actually our very first line of defense. We are hard-wired to seek safety first by reaching out to others for social connection (Porges & Furman, 2011). For your child, this means that his first response to any stress is to reach out to you!

This reaching out response begins at birth when the mother touches her baby and the baby turns to face her and make eye contact. A mother's touch in that moment activates a flood of positive signals in both their bodies that calm the heart and turn on this other system, the relax-and-relate mode. This creates, quite literally, a 'touch-face-heart connection' between you and your child, making the two of you open, alert and fully receptive to each other. When relax-and-relate works, your child feels safe, which instantly dials down the fight-flight-or-freeze part of the brain. As you will see in the next chapter, a maturing relax-and-relate mode provides the building blocks for all future positive behavior and for social, emotional and mental growth.

A Sensory Solution

We began this chapter with the dilemma for parents – that your natural attempts to soothe through touch or words can often result in the exact opposite of what you intend. And that focusing on controlling or trying to fix the behavior may only over-stimulate and exacerbate your child's feeling of overwhelm. You now know that the root of the problem is *not his behavior*, and the goal is to go *underneath* the behaviors to the sensory overload causing them. The key to doing that is the guidance you can provide through your skilled and attuned touch because *sensory problems respond best to sensory solutions*.

QST is sensory treatment that focuses on helping your child's nervous system move into the relax-relate mode and, over time, ingraining that ability so he can calm and regulate all on his own. The daily routine offers an organized approach to both stimulating and calming the senses. And that also depends on the little things: your reassuring facial expression, the tone of your voice and, as you will see in the following chapters, especially on your attuned and skilled touch – one of your most effective therapeutic tools. Each daily repetition of the QST routine helps condition your child's nervous system so that he can be more receptive to the touch-face-heart connection with you. Your attunement to his body and behavioral cues as you do QST is the key to helping your child reach this open and receptive place.

Bibliography

Chapter 1

Hopkins, Susan (2016). *The Journey of Self-Reg Learning*, The MEHRIT Centre, Peterborough, ON, Canada, [The Journey of Learning Self-Reg Video].

Porges, S.W., & Furman, S.A. (2011). The early development of the autonomic nervous system provides a neural platform for social behavior: A polyvagal perspective. *Infant and Child Development*, 20(1), 106–118.

Shanker, Stuart (2016). *Self-Reg: How to Help Your Child (and You) Break the Stress Cycle and Successfully Engage with Life*, Penguin Random House, New York, NY.

Suggested Readings

Brain-Body Parenting: How to Stop Managing Behavior and Start Raising Joyful, Resilient Kids, by Mona Delahooke, (2022) Harper Wave, an Imprint of HarperCollins Publishers, New York.

The Child with Special Needs: Encouraging Intellectual and Emotional Growth, by Stanley Greenspan, M.D. & Serena Weider, Ph.D., (1998) Perseus Books, Reading, MA.

The Explosive Child, by Ross Green, (2021) Harper Collins Publishers, New York.

No Longer A Secret: Unique Common Sense Strategies for Children with Sensory and Regulation Challenges (2nd ed.), by Lucy Jane Miller, Lisa M. Porter & Doreit S. Bialer, (2021) Arlington, TX: Future Horizons, USA.

The Whole-Brain Child: 12 Revolutionary Strategies to Nurture Your Child's Developing Mind, by Daniel J. Siegel & Tina Payne Bryson, (2012) Delacorte Press, Random House, New York.

Chapter 2

Self-Regulation – A Parent's Gift

At the time I started QST my son was not sleeping well. He had some spectacular tantrums that could last for what seemed like forever. I used to call him my Ferrari because he could go from 0–60 in a few seconds. Food was another challenge. He was a very fussy eater. He was having a very difficult time adjusting to school. He was hitting the staff and I was worried he would be thrown out of school. He had many sensory challenges – hypersensitive to light, sound and some touch (he wouldn't wear socks).

At the end of the five months he was wearing socks, tantrums were less frequent both at home and at school, he was sleeping much better and had even started playing around with words to make simple jokes! Two years later, we still do QST several times a week.

Mother of a 4-year-old

Children aren't born knowing how to behave; they learn this first from you. But when your child is in survival mode, it is difficult for them to take in even the most caring guidance and support from you, other caregivers or teachers. Sensory children's immature nervous systems are easily and frequently triggered into sensory overload; it takes them much longer to calm down, and even when they do, they often don't stay that way for long. This repeated inability to take in support and guidance disrupts a child's ability to achieve what we term the 'basic self-regulation developmental milestones', which shape her ability to experience and organize her own feelings and behaviors. Without this foundation, social and learning delays almost always occur. In this chapter, we take a closer look at what these self-regulation milestones are, why they are so important and what happens to a child if she misses one or more of them. Then we'll show you how QST's organizing sensory messages can help to mature the sensory nervous system's responses and, in turn, help your child reach milestones she may have missed. As these milestones are achieved, you can expect to see increased awareness, reduced reactivity and greater ease in regulating behavior.

We've found that parents' eyes often glaze over when we mention 'self-regulation milestones', so we need to start by taking a closer look at development in the first year of life. While the term sounds complicated, the idea is pretty basic. Let's start with a few questions to point us in the right direction:

Do I want my child to sleep through the night? Yes, definitely!
Do I want her to be less picky with foods? Please!
Do I want the constipation and diarrhea to stop? Absolutely!

DOI: 10.4324/9781003360421-4

Do I want the tantrums to stop? Of course!

Do I want her to make eye contact and pay attention? I would love that!

Each of these – sleeplessness, pickiness with food, digestive regularity, tantrums and attention issues – are examples of problems relating to one of the *four basic self-regulation milestones* that every child needs to grow:

1. Regular sleep – being a good sleeper
2. Regular digestion – being a good eater with good appetite/digestion/elimination
3. The ability pay attention – being a good learner, making easy transitions
4. The ability to self-soothe – able to deal with daily ups and downs

Most parents are keenly tuned in to the basic growth milestones that you and your pediatrician watch for. Is your baby rolling over from back to tummy at three months, sitting up with assistance by six months, crawling by nine months? What percentile are they for height or weight? Physical growth milestones help us to identify and chart those skills that must be achieved for a child to reach physical maturity. With Louisa's insight, we can understand the building blocks of self-regulation in much the same way, focusing not on *physical* growth but on your child's growing capacity to regulate and manage all aspects of her body, mind, feelings and behavior. And that all begins with you!

A Parent's Gift of Regulation

When everything is going well in those first years of life, a baby's capacity for self-regulation develops naturally through repeated soothing. Your baby is totally dependent on you to calm and regulate her upsets and discomforts. Each time you soothe her, you learn what works best for her while she learns that she can rely on you to keep her safe. This back-and-forth process repeats over and over again, building in her a sense of trust that her upsets will be calmed by you. This connection with you is her *first line of defense against stress*. The feel of your touch, the calming sound of your voice, a yummy meal and your loving gaze all help to organize and regulate your baby's initial experiences and feelings and, most importantly, turn off the need for those survival-mode reactions.

Over time, it is this connection and regulating interaction with you that strengthens and matures her nervous system responses as she begins to learn that being stressed does not have to signal a survival risk. The sense of order and safety you provide gives her the blueprint she will use to get back to that place of calm, open receptivity on her own. Her behavior becomes more organized and her emotions more stable. This growing ability to self-regulate or return to calm is a journey that is achieved step-by-step and is measured by the self-regulation milestones in these important first years. Let's take a look at each milestone and how they build on one another.

The Self-Regulation Milestones – Four Pillars of Health

The four Early Self-Regulation Milestones, as represented in Figure 2.1, set the foundation for good health. The first two, good sleep and digestion, provide the physical foundation for growth. The next two, which revolve around the ability to calm down, focus and pay attention, provide the foundation for language, thinking, behavior and social connection. When everything is going

Early Self-Regulation Milestones [1]

Healthy development depends on a child's ability to achieve these
early self-regulation milestones in the first years of life.

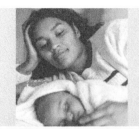

Regulated Sleep

Consistent parent-co-regulated routines help build an inner self-
regulated self-wake cycle that the child comes to own for herself.

Regulated Appetite & Digestion

Parents set the stage for healthy digestion and regulated
patterns of appetite, feeding and elimination.

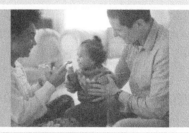

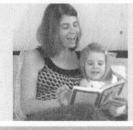

Orientation & Attention

The self-regulation of orientation and attention is the starting
point for social learning and sets the stage for being a good
learner and making easy transitions.

Capacity to Self-Soothe

The capacity to be soothed, and in turn learn to self-
soothe, comes from repeated co-regulation with
parent(s).

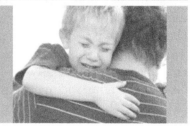

**A parent's touch and co-regulation help children
to activate and achieve these milestones.**

Regulated sleep and digestion provide the foundation for physical growth.

The capacities to pay attention and self-soothe provide the foundation
for emotional, social and cognitive growth, and language development.

Figure 2.1 **Early Self-Regulation Milestones** — by Louisa Silva, MD, Qigong Sensory Training
Institute.

well, all of the milestones are activated and achieved through a parent's touch and 'co-regulating' influence.

1. Regulation of the Sleep/Wake Cycle

Soon after birth, parents help set their baby's regulatory clock. The hundreds and thousands of times they rhythmically rock, hold and soothe and the many times they let the baby fall asleep on their body (whole-body touch) and let them stay there all provide the necessary elements – safety, warmth, comfort and predictability – that help the baby achieve regulated sleep. This consistent parent-regulated routine helps the baby build an inner self-regulated sleep/wake cycle that she comes to own for herself.

2. Regulation of Appetite and Digestion

A child achieves regulated appetite and digestion through the thousands of times that she is held, fed on a regular schedule, burped and changed when uncomfortable. Parents make sure there is a variety of healthy and appropriate foods that are adjusted to meet her needs. This ability to provide predictability, mixed with sensitive attunement to discomfort, sets the 'digestive clock' that helps the child 'tick' with regularity. In these ways, the parent sets the stage for healthy digestion and regulated patterns of appetite, feeding and elimination.

3. Regulation of Orientation and Focused Attention

Attention begins with your touch, which sends signals to your child's brain stem, where all the necessary nerves originate together, ready and hard-wired to receive your signal. That touch triggers an intricate process – her heart rate slows, her body movements quiet, she turns to face you, focuses her eyes on your eyes, attunes her ears to your voice and connects with you in open, focused receptivity. This seemingly simple but miraculous sequence is where all attention begins, on you! It begins at birth when you and your baby meet in that first magical loving gaze, where connection and attention first become one.

When all goes well, this focused attention matures and strengthens through nursing and in all the thousands of ways that you responded positively, as you care for and play with her in those first years. She becomes more adept at making eye contact and listening for your voice as you teach her to imitate *your* sounds by imitating hers. Connecting and responding comes to feel good, so she practices it with you and the rest of the family. As she practices and you guide her toward a receptive state, she learns that paying attention and maintaining focus can be fun and rewarding. Her skills mature and the foundation gets set for her to direct her own attention for longer and longer periods of time, first with you, then with others and later at school and in the world – all by herself.

4. The Capacity to Be Soothed and to Self-Soothe

By picking up and soothing your child when she is upset, her nervous system learns how to calm down. As she comes to understand that you will consistently be there to soothe her, she learns trust which, in itself, is soothing. With this basis of trust and consistency and with your continued co-regulation to fall back on, she discovers the ways that she can soothe herself, and those patterns become ingrained in her brain and body. At first, she may suck on her fingers, rock herself or cuddle a favorite stuffed toy. As she gets older, she may insist that you read to her, or she may sing herself a lullaby. She soon finds that she can control the level of her upset and reduce the time it takes her to come back to a calmer state.

We are born with a highly active survival mode (sympathetic nervous system), but we have to build our relax-and-relate system through this repeated co-regulation, re-regulation and support. For a child, achieving the relax-and-relate mode on her own is a major developmental accomplishment. Once this response is more developed, she will be able to calm herself down when distress triggers her fears, even without her parent present. While this ability to self-soothe may sound like a fairly basic childhood skill, it is the basis of virtually all self-regulation and mature, goal-based behavior in every adult. The child with effective strategies to self-soothe can grow into an adult who can respond to life's ups and downs without undue disruption. While there will always be stressors to face, she will not get stuck in either extreme for too long because she has learned how to find her own way back to recover, rest and restore.

As you can see, self-regulation is not just a matter of self-control. It is *what children need to make self-control possible*. Together, these four milestones provide that foundation by establishing a broad and essential range of capacities from the most basic of biological functions (sleep and digestion) to much more mature abilities (maintaining attention and self-soothing). Like a wide umbrella, self-regulation provides the basis for your child's ability to manage and balance her body, feelings and behaviors. When all goes well, she learns to calm herself in the face of frustration, finds ways to socially express displeasure without exploding and (as the old saying goes) 'plays well with others'. Her sensory triggers and reactivity mature over time, so she can flexibly meet the environment without becoming avoidant or over-reactive.

The ability to achieve all of this is hard-wired in most of us and, as we will see in the next chapter, it is a parent's loving touch that plays the central role in this back and forth between being regulated and self-regulation. Children learn to regulate themselves through a slow and patient dance between the parent's ability to be responsive in one moment and provide guidance in the next. It starts from the bottom of the biological cycle, with touch, and works its way up to feeling and thinking.

While most of this self-regulatory learning and growth happens naturally as a parent's regulatory guidance and support is taken in through the senses, when a child's sensory apparatus is impaired, problems can arise and this virtuous circle can be blocked. A child with sensory difficulties is like a hungry baby who can't take in that sensory food. You could say that sensory data doesn't quite 'taste good' because it is coming in slightly distorted, muted or overly harsh. The result is a child who can't absorb the parent's natural efforts to soothe, feed or regulate and so is stuck in survival mode. As a result, the four pillars of self-regulation cannot fully mature, causing the underlying sensory under- or over-reactivity to intensify, along with the meltdowns and anxieties. And, if these self-regulatory milestones are not achieved by the age of three, any child will have problems regulating both her emotions and her behavior.

Finding a Way Back to Growth

Fortunately, children are amazingly resilient. You may be surprised to know that even as she is struggling, fidgeting or pushing you away, your child will be your partner. Children have a strong innate sense of what they need in order to grow. While they can't express it verbally, their body cues and behaviors will show you the way. But, as you can imagine, it will require some effort on your part to learn to get 'under' your child's over-sensitive radar so you can help her become receptive to her surroundings and your helpful regulatory patterns. And you will not be working alone; QST will teach you that certain of her signals mean 'stop' while others mean 'I need more of this'. And as your ability to read and respond to her cues increases, you will find that your child has even greater resilience to heal herself. That's because once you free her from sensory stress mode, your child has the marvelous capacity to naturally go back and restore the missed milestones with your co-regulating support. Sleep and digestion often improve first. Then you will see changes in attention and the ability to regulate feelings and behavior.

Once freed from their survival mode, it's almost like children naturally go back to pick up the steps in development that they missed along the way. Children just naturally do this. Our job is to give them the chance. In the next chapter, we'll show you how guided touch provides a road map into your child's brain pathways. It restores receptivity and improves sensory and behavior problems so that your child can go back and reclaim those self-regulation milestones that she missed and so desperately needs.

Chapter 3

Attuned Touch – Your Sensory Solution

We know from Chapter 1 that *sensory problems require a sensory solution*. But it is easy for parents to under-estimate just how important positive touch is for healthy growth and how effective their own touch can be for improving their child's sensory and behavior problems. Children with sensory issues have many roadblocks that make it hard for them to find a place of calm, open receptivity. For a child with sensory problems, touch signals can come into the brain in ways that create a confusing stressful experience that triggers survival mode. To reach the root of your child's sensory reactivity, we need to chart a direct path *below* language and behavior, all the way back to the developmental beginnings of the senses themselves. And, of all the senses, none develop earlier in life or are more fundamental to your child's healthy development than touch. Our understanding of the roots and treatment of sensory and behavioral problems centers on this one sense. Touch sits at the very base of a huge developmental pyramid. Alter touch and you impact all development that subsequently takes place above it.

The types of touch that children receive in the womb and in the earliest hours, days and years of life create the basic neural networks for future growth and development. The neurons for our senses of touch, balance (vestibular system), where our body is in space (proprioception), and our inner body signals (interoception) provide these underlying foundational circuits (see Figure 3.1). All future neural connections for brain development, awareness and learning are built upon these early sensory links. This means that all awareness and learning starts in the body. Development, behavior and self-regulation are all built upon on these early connections.

However, touch tends to be a forgotten area because our modern culture has ignored and even unwittingly rejected the importance of a parent's touch for a child's healthy development. Yet for centuries, grandmothers have known just how important it is. In most traditional cultures around the world, daily rhythmic touch routines have been handed down from grandmother to new mother through the generations. In many African, Indian and Asian cultures, the grandmother gives the new baby a daily massage for the first 40 days of life while the new mother watches, learns and, in some cultures, gets a massage from *her* mother or aunts. After 40 days, the mother takes over the daily massage for her own baby. This time-honored tradition supports good development and bonding, addresses the baby's sensory needs, and naturally provides a foundation for the achievement of those all-important early self-regulatory milestones.

Traditional cultures followed this path because grandmothers instinctively knew the fundamental connection between their touch and their children's healthy growth. They knew that this was exactly what their babies needed to sleep better, eat better, get along better and grow up

DOI: 10.4324/9781003360421-5

Pyramid of Learning

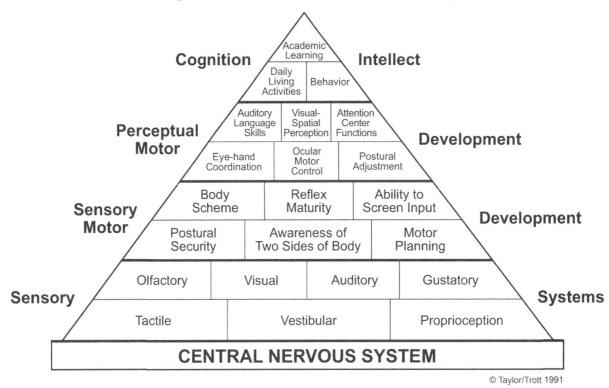

Figure 3.1 **The Pyramid of Learning** – touch sits at the base of an organized and orderly development. Each skill or capacity is built upon those that came before.

Source: Reproduced with permission from AlertProgram.com from their online course & textbook. (Taylor & Trott 1991)

stronger. Modern science now confirms what grandmothers have known for centuries, that touch is the earliest and most central path for shaping and informing all bonding and development. And *without* proper touch, this natural path can go terribly wrong. For example, in institutions where children have not been given caring touch, their bodies and minds actually stop growing. Yet once they are placed with families where they receive positive touch through a loving relationship, the damage can begin to be repaired and their bodies and minds start growing again. While such extreme experiences don't apply to your own child, they do show us how critical the simple act of caring touch is for all children, especially in the early years when the brain is growing the fastest. Touch is essential to life itself. Children need it like plants need the sun. A child can thrive without the sense of hearing or vision but he cannot survive without nurturing touch (Field, 2010; Thompson, 2016).

> *Social touch is a powerful force in human development, shaping social reward, attachment, cognitive, communication, and emotional regulation from infancy and throughout life.*
>
> (Cascio et al., 2019)

Of all the senses, touch offers two unique features that can help you reach your child through even the most difficult sensory obstacles. First, it is wired directly to the brain through its own special neural pathway, so when you touch your child's skin, your attuned touch signal goes directly to the parts of his brain where it can do the most good and turn off the stress response. Secondly, that link provides, as no other sense does, simultaneous two-way feedback. Think about it – you can see without being seen. You can hear without being heard. But *you cannot touch without being touched* in return. Only this sense gives and receives a signal *at the same time*, so you can feel your child's reactions and adjust to them instantaneously. Your touch becomes the medicine that provides a direct route to the brain while carrying a free-flowing, back-and-forth channel of communication. It's the perfect pathway to our sensory solution.

The touch-brain connection

In the embryo, the skin and the central nervous system are the first to develop. In fact, they are formed from the same outer layer of embryonic tissue. That layer folds in on itself, creating the central nervous system on the inside and the skin on the outside.

Among the first neurons to wire together are those for touch sensations in the skin, along with neurons responsible for our awareness of our body position, movement, balance and inner body sensations. These neurons and connections form the base from which all future brain development happens. So, you can think of the *skin as the external portion of the nervous system*, with a direct pathway to the brain.

A Special Touch Highway

Nerve endings just under the skin's surface are literally one synapse (a single nerve connection) away from the self-regulating systems in your child's brain. With the right kind of organizing touch, this network of connections creates a sensory highway that guides you right to the heart of his over-reactive stress response. We are all familiar with how instantaneously we pull away when we touch something too hot. Those nerve signals travel so quickly from your skin to your brain that you react even before you can think about it. They are carried on fast-acting fibers that register sensations like temperature, pain, itch, pressure and vibration to give us instantaneous feedback. These pathways are well known. However, in recent years, neuroscientists have discovered that under this huge highway of fast-acting sensory nerves lies an entirely different roadway of touch fibers that focus specifically on pleasurable touch, the kind that parents use in attachment and bonding (Fairhurst et al., 2022; Cascio et al., 2019; McGlone, 2014). These touch signals travel along their very own set of nerves, which scientists call 'C-tactile fibers'. This type of pleasurable touch is so important that it has its own separate wiring and is processed in a unique and special way in the brain.

Unlike the fast-acting touch signals that, by necessity, must travel rapidly to the brain and allow us to react quickly, pleasurable touch signals travel more slowly along the C-tactile fibers. Marching to a different beat, they are attuned to the slower rhythms that convey nurturing affection, such as those between parent and child. Most importantly, these fibers relay nurturing touch signals directly to the more primitive parts of the brain, where they can turn off stress alarms in an immature sensory nervous system stuck in high-alert survival mode. But what truly sets the

C-tactile highway apart from the fast-acting fibers is that their signals are also processed in the area of the brain responsible for emotions, bonding and behavior. This means that C-fibers signal more than just sensations, they convey the *feelings of pleasure* and the *safety of social contact*. This is a powerful combination that delivers the very signals of security that turn off fight-flight-or-freeze and open your child to social connection (Brummelman, 2019).

While they travel on their own highway, C-tactile fibers work in concert with the fast-acting fibers, adding true dimension to the experience of touch. This vast highway of tactile fibers helps to create an important boundary between ourselves and the outside world. The skin is where we stop and the world begins, and that boundary helps us to know who we are and where we are in relation to others. When touch fiber signals travel from the skin to the somatosensory area of your child's brain, they create a complete picture or sensory 'map' of our body. This map gives us our sense of self, where we are in space and how all of the parts of our body fit together as a whole (Blakeslee & Blakeslee, 2007). Touch is 'hard-wired' to create this organized picture of the body within the brain. We understand our other senses in an integrated way through this map, and when sensory impairments render that map incomplete, it can result in problems in overall development, including that of motor, social and learning skills.

From Safety to Growth

The key to helping the child begin to move back to a more regulated state, making the child feel safe and thereby more available for cognitive engagement and therapeutic change, is to utilize the direct so-matosensory routes and provide patterned, repetitive, rhythmic input. Therapeutic change starts from a sense of safety in turn, the sense of safety emerges from these regulating somatosensory activities.

Bruce D. Perry, MD (Gaskill & Perry, 2014)

Think of your touch like food for the brain. Every time you hold, rock or care for your child, millions of tiny sensory nerves in the skin are activated, sending messages that affect bonding, body awareness (Montirosso & McGlone, 2020), immunity, attention, motor control, emotional maturity and a host of other vital capacities and skills. You and your child create a powerful circuit that flows along the special touch-fiber highways and allows you direct access to your child's survival brain, his emotional brain and his sensory body map.

Your touch has the amazing ability to turn down his stress alarms, convey affection and bring order, rhythm and predictability to his sensory confusion so you can guide him to the receptive calm mode where he feels safe and is ready to meet the world. These form the foundation for all learning, growth and development to take place. But attuned touch does much more. Through the unique properties of the skin and its porous yet protective boundary to the outside world, attuned touch awakens circuits in the brain necessary for complex motor skills, emotions and communication. Let's take a closer look at these hidden treasures.

Body awareness and motor skills. Touch creates body awareness, which is essential for the development of good motor skills. Because it comes so naturally, we often don't appreciate how our touch shapes this internal body map and initiates the direct connection to the motor part of the brain. An organized and integrated body map helps us feel oriented and allows us to more fully learn and coordinate motor movements.

Think about those first moments after birth. When you touch your baby's face, you wake up the motor part of his brain that initiates his turning to face you. When you stroke down his neck and back, you wake up the muscles that help him learn to lift his head and hold his back straight. And when you play with his fingers, you activate and guide the circuits that help him learn to point and then develop finer and finer movements, like writing or using a scissors.

Through the early years, it is your touch that shapes more and more complex motor skills and gives them social meaning. That's because *how* we point, *where* we walk and *how* we move are as much social as they are physical acts. So, when you touch your child's skin, you are not only triggering a movement circuit but also gradually guiding, bringing order, focus and social meaning to that movement. It is that combination that makes all the difference between your child merely making random movements and his engaging in socially organized motor skills.

Emotional development. Just as motor skills are awakened and then shaped by a parent's touch, so too are healthy and regulated emotions. Children's feelings are body-based and can get held in their muscles and tissues. When you touch your child, you make a connection that directly touches his emotions. The right kind of touch can help him to process and even release those emotions that get 'stuck inside' because they are too scary, painful or complicated to deal with on his own.

If your toddler falls on the playground and hurts himself, he needs to be held and soothed until he calms down. When you touch or simply hold him, you bypass words and gestures and go directly to his body where his feelings are stored. This not only triggers the release of calming 'feel good' hormones, it also awakens the body-brain circuit for the relax-and-restore mode. When that occurs, your child is open to your emotional guidance. At this point, your sensitive touch can literally 'guide' his emotions toward responses that are more appropriate to his needs and the distressing situation. If nobody is there to hold and soothe him, he'll eventually calm down, but he won't have a way to process the upset either physically or emotionally. And then, the next time he is on the playground, he is more likely to be fearful or anxious. It is through this continuous feedback that you give shape to his confused emotions so he can go back to playing and feel unafraid. Over time, he'll learn to develop those soothing and regulating skills his own.

Touch, movement and emotions are all closely related for children. When we forget this and then don't make use of the benefits of touch, it's easy to turn to other means of comforting that at best only help in the moment. For example, it might seem natural to try to soothe your child's emotions by using food or by putting him in front of the TV when he is upset. But feeding a child when he is not hungry does not help him process the source of the upset. Neither will distracting a child with TV. This is not to say that you can't use them, but while these diversions may calm your child in the moment, they won't help his ability to regulate in the future. When anxious and lacking the ability to self-soothe, he may turn to food or electronic games instead of seeking more restorative forms of support and reassurance.

Communication skills. Touch, with its unique, instantaneous two-way exchange, is our first means of communication. It starts in the first moments after birth, when you touch his face and he turns to make eye contact. This connection is his first milestone in communication, the earliest form of 'non-verbal' conversation. He then learns to communicate by smiling and making noises and you respond by imitating his response. In time, he comes to understand that this is a two-way street and that he has the power to get you to respond positively. This back-and-forth exchange is his blueprint for all future spoken language and reassures him that communication can be safe and pleasurable. Over time, as you listen and respond to his cues in attuned ways through your 'language of touch', he comes to understand the 'rhythm' of conversation and that listening and respect are what help it to grow.

For children who have problems with listening, communication and relatedness, we often need to go back to the very beginning, to the 'language of touch', to re-learn the steps of the dance through direct experience. Through your daily QST time together, you will create moments where your child, whether verbal or non-verbal, becomes intensely interested in communicating with you. Over the years, many parents have reported to us how their non-expressive child has opened up and talked about their feelings or fears during the routine. To some parents, this seems like magic. But the answer is simple. With QST to guide you, your intentional touch lays down new and healthy patterns of communication and reciprocity, opening the doors that have felt locked and inaccessible.

When I pick Maggie up from school and ask her how her day was she only shrugs. It's only once we start doing our QST at night that, on her own, she opens up and begins to tell me all about what happened during her day. It's one of our favorite times together.

Mother of a 6-year-old

Empathy. A final unseen treasure that touch holds is the gift of empathy itself. The unique thing about empathy is that, just like touch, its essence is reciprocal: we cannot have true empathy for others unless we have empathy for ourselves. Through empathy, we emotionally touch another as we ourselves are touched. It begins with our body awareness, which scaffolds a sense of self that allows us, over time, to really feel *for* and *with* another. Mature and reciprocal empathy is our highest achievement as human beings. To understand its sources, we can picture it as sitting at the pinnacle of a large pyramid of learned and earned skills and capabilities. Much like the Pyramid of Learning in Figure 3.1 (page 28), that ability to feel others rests on a number of fundamentals – the inner map of our bodies, our sensory and body awareness, motor skills, emotional development and communication skills. Those skills themselves are based on a foundation of touch which, in its humble ability to turn off stress alarms, conveys affection and brings organization to experience, forming the foundation for the ever-growing capacities that arise from it.

A Heart-to-Heart Connection

With touch, you have the perfect highway to all areas of healthy development because the feedback from your child to you is immediate and your reactions can attune to his with exquisite sensitivity. Your sensory child does not even need to be verbal. You can feel, through your two-way touch, when he is dysregulated, uncomfortable or overwhelmed. You can react immediately to soothe and give the sense of safety that he needs at that precise moment. As you help him to regulate, again and again, you make his world predictable and literally show him what it feels like to be calm. He learns what a sense of peace feels like because you take him there. You awaken the necessary brain circuits and guide him to more mature ways of responding. You help him define his boundaries in space and create an integrated inner map of his own body. This is really how infants learn to regulate themselves. It is the basis for achieving all the early self-regulation milestones we talked about and, in the end, for helping him build the capacities to master and regulate his feelings and behaviors.

With this new knowledge and with the help of the QST movements to guide your touch and sharpen your intuition, you can do all this and much more. Your own inner intention, your feelings and your skilled touch are what make all the difference. *The link goes heart-to-heart, intention-to-intention and calm-to-calm.* When you combine this with the reassuring tone of your voice and the warm expression on your face, all the planets align for getting your child back to a calm, connected and receptive state, no matter what the upset.

Bibliography

Chapter 3

Blakeslee, S., & Blakeslee, M. (2007). *The Body has a Mind of Its Own: How Body Maps in Your Brain Help You Do (Almost) Everything Better*, Random House Inc., New York, 4–27.

Brummelman, E., Terburg, D., Smit, M., Bögels, S.M., & Bos, P.A. (2019). Parental touch reduces social vigilance in children. *Developmental Cognitive Neuroscience*, 35, 87–93.

Cascio, C.J., Moore, D., & McGlone, F. (2019). Social touch and human development. *Developmental Cognitive Neuroscience*, 35, 5–11.

Fairhurst, M.T., McGlone, F., & Croy, I. (2022). Affective touch: A communication channel for social exchange. *Current Opinion in Behavioral Sciences*, 43, 54–61.

Field, T. (2010). Touch for socioemotional and physical well-being: A review. *Developmental Review*, 30(4), 367–383.

Gaskill, R.L., & Perry, B.D. (2014). The neurobiological power of play: Using the neurosequential model of therapeutics to guide play in the healing process. In C.A. Malchiodi, & D.A. Crenshaw (Eds.), *Creative Arts and Play Therapy for Attachment Problems*, The Guilford Press, New York, 178–194.

McGlone, F., Wessberg, J., & Olausson, H. (2014). Discriminative and affective touch: Sensing and feeling. *Neuron*, 82(4), 737–755.

Montirosso, R., & McGlone, F. (2020). The body comes first. Embodied reparation and the co-creation of infant bodily-self. *Neuroscience & Biobehavioral Reviews*, 113, 77–87.

Taylor, K., & Trott, M. (1991) in Williams, M.S., & Shellenberger, S. (1996). *"How Does Therapy-Works, Inc. ©2022 Copyright Guidelines for TherapyWorks, Inc. Last Updated 7/19/22 11 Your Engine Run?"® A Leader's Guide to the Alert Program® for Self-Regulation*, TherapyWorks, Inc., Albuquerque, NM.

Thompson, E.H. (2016). The effects of touch. In H. Olausson, J. Wessberg, I. Morrison, & F. McGlone (Eds.), *Affective Touch and the Neurophysiology of CT Afferents*, Springer, New York, NY, 341–353.

Suggested Readings

Books:

Affective Touch and the Neurophysiology of CT Afferents, Edited by H. Olausson, J. Wessberg, I. Morrison & F.P. McGlone, (2016) Springer, New York.

Essential Touch: Meeting the Needs of Young Children, by Frances M. Carlson, (2006) NAEYC, Washington, DC.

The Handbook of Touch: Neuroscience, Behavioral and Health Perspectives, Edited by M. Hertenstein &
 S.J. Weiss, (2011) Springer, New York.
Touch, by Tiffany Field, (2001) Bradford Book, MIT Press, Cambridge, MA.
Touch in Child Counseling and Play Therapy: An Ethical and Clinical Guide, Edited by Janet A. Court-
 ney & Robert D. Nolan, (2017) Routledge, New York.
Touching: The Human Significance of the Skin (3rd ed.), by Ashley Montagu, (1986) Perennial Library,
 Harper and Row, New York.

Article:

The social power of touch, by Lydia Denworth, (2015) *Scientific Mind*, July/August, 30–39.

Chapter 4

QST – A Sensory Language

When I started QST I thought, this is impossible. How can patting the skin help? But then I learned how to do it and realized it's just so natural, it's the kind of touch that works and it's what we do anyway.

Mother of a 4-year-old

Over the years we've found that some parents want to know more about how and why QST works. How can my touch actually make changes in my child's sensory and behavior problems? What's actually happening when I do QST? How can simply patting and pressing affect the brain? Understanding how we change is never easy. And for children with sensory and self-regulation problems and their related behavioral difficulties, the problems feel even more mysterious and inaccessible. But new approaches to age-old problems often come from the creative mix of very different perspectives, and it's here that Louisa came to this task well prepared. Her training and experience in Chinese medicine offered the key, a different way to look at and treat sensory difficulties.

The Eastern perspective does not see sensory difficulties only as a problem of the brain and central nervous system. It focuses on the whole child, her entire body and the flow of energy throughout it. That means that the outer edges of the nervous system, at the periphery, can be just as important as the brain itself. That insight inspired Louisa to expand her original research focus to include a relatively neglected neural area, that vast set of nerve fibers found at the surface of the skin that bring sensory information from the outside world back to the brain for processing. And with this simple shift in perspective began years of autism research confirming the key role that these peripheral nerves and the sense of touch play in all sensory, attentional and regulatory problems.

Changing the Perspective

It was a radical shift of focus with many important implications for how we understand sensory problems, how we treat them, who can treat them and, finally, how we connect them to the development of self-regulation skills. And it all started with Louisa's insight that parent touch plays a key role. That insight opened a doorway for her to use the language of the senses as a means of real two-way communication between a parent and a child with regulation difficulties. And it gave us a way to offer, through QST, *a sensory solution to children's sensory, self-regulation and related behavioral problems.*

DOI: 10.4324/9781003360421-6

So, what's happening when a child is so easily vulnerable to being overwhelmed? In Chinese medicine, we can say that the child's 'sensory doors close'. Or, from a Western perspective, that the sensory triggers and thresholds are too under- or over-reactive. Or, from an evolutionary angle, that the survival-mode stress response is constantly jammed on. All of these metaphors point to an out-of-balance reactivity to sensory input that is stuck in a cycle that cascades first into emotional and behavioral disruptions and later into social and learning problems.

Knowing this, it's tempting to conclude that the solution is simply to calm your child so that she will be more open and receptive to you and her environment. But calming your child, even if you can repeatedly get her to relax, doesn't guarantee that she will be able to open those doors to connection and experience *whenever she really needs to*. She first has to experience from *you* what it *feels* like to have those doors open and to experience the feeling of her body and mind becoming calm. Then, with each daily repetition of QST, the organized sensory 'messages' you send from her skin to her brain help her 'own' that relaxed and open state. And your touch helps her immature sensory nervous system move to a more integrated, mature and higher-order level of organization. Slowly and over time, this builds inner capacities for self-regulation so that when her sensory alarms are triggered, she now has a new 'template' in her brain and nervous system with which to shift back into the more comfortable relax-and-relate mode, all on her own.

Opening the Sensory Doors

Chinese medicine defines this problem as one in which the 'sensory doors have closed'. For a parent whose child is overwhelmed by her environment, this definition may seem exactly back-ward. Their child's sensory doors don't feel closed; they probably feel precariously wide-open to the world. But that kind of unintegrated openness leads to disorganization and overwhelm that can cascade into behavioral problems. The over- or under-reactivity of the nervous system actu-ally leaves them 'closed off' from much of the opportunity for the calming and connected sensa-tions necessary for growth. But looked at through an Eastern lens where the goal of openness is to foster organization of the senses and regulated behavior, we see a different picture. Here, open sensory doors are associated with a capacity to organize and make sense of the information com-ing in from the world, and that can only happen when there is a state of relaxed, open receptivity which fosters the ability to engage with and relate to others.

For that to occur, your child needs to learn that opening those sensory doors to the outer world will leave her feeling entirely safe. Without that, nothing can change. But even that is only the first step. Being made to feel safe, even learning and trusting that there is safety to be gained by relaxing your guard, is not the same as being able to internalize and attain that sense of safety from within. Your child needs the inner resources to navigate her way back to that place when things get out of balance. Safety only sets the stage for the more difficult and important challenge: to learn that in the end, she can finally rely on her inner capacities to get to that place of safety and regulation from within herself.

That inner ability to shift to a place of calm and safety can't be imposed from the outside. Your child needs to learn it from you through direct experience as you take her there. And that's what QST does – it places you on the C-tactile fiber highway to deliver the *organizing sensory mes-sages* and feelings of safety to the exact place in her brain and body that will turn off the sensory alarms and turn on the relax-relate-receptive mode. When this is repeated day after day, over and over, you not only take your child to that calm, open receptive place but you help her 'learn' those regulation skills for herself, right in her bones. It is a uniquely intimate regulatory/organizational process that takes place both between you and your child and *within* her at the same time. It may all sound very complex, but with the right touch and QST skills, it can really be quite simple.

Think of your child as an immature driver sitting at the controls of a fast car – her own body and emotions – that she doesn't yet have the skills to control. When you try to only control her behavior, you are like a traffic cop trying to direct her erratic driving from the outside. You can set rules and put up stop signs or even roadblocks, but your impact is limited because you are outside her body looking in. Now imagine you can get *inside* the car as her co-pilot. Think of one of those driving school cars with a separate set of controls. Touch's unique qualities give you this same kind of direct access to establish an organized connection between her brain and all the sensory information coming in from the outside world. It lets you not only get inside her world but also communicate with her through touch – the sensory language of the body – that it is now safe to open the sensory doors.

A Sensory Language

The sensory language in QST begins by communicating with two very simple 'touch messages', patting and pressing. These two touch techniques, which you will learn in Chapters 7 and 8, involve your skilled alternating between quick patting movements and slower deeper pressing movements. Patting is done more rapidly and with a relaxed cupped hand, while the slower rhythmic pressing movements use the full surface of your hands and the warmth of your palms to bring calm. As you learn to skillfully switch between these two techniques, you send touch signals that convey you will respond with just the right touch that she needs at exactly the moment when she needs it. You'll learn to communicate that information through how you shift your touch based on your child's cues – how and when you shift from patting to pressing, where you linger on a certain spot or how you use more or less pressure, all in response to her body and behavioral cues. It develops into a naturally flowing back-and-forth conversation.

You can think of when and how you pat and press as a kind of Morse code that you send, one that your child's body knows how to 'read' without even having to decode. Each choice and shift that you make in response to your child's cues shows her and lets her feel what an organized sensory response to her frightened cues might look and feel like. You'll be surprised at how much just shifting between patting and pressing can tell your child in this simple way. For example, if you see your child wince and bend her ear toward her shoulder when you pat around the ear, you will switch to a slower deeper pressing. That switch 'tells' her that you see her discomfort and are responding to the stress response that your patting ignited. By adapting your touch, you will now guide her back to feelings of safety and calm.

With that message, you lend your child a kind of co-regulated first step toward self-regulation, one that comes from both the outside and the inside at the same time. That regulation, as we've said in previous chapters, all starts with a more clearly defined and integrated body map taking shape in your child's brain, a map shaped and organized by the sensory signals you send with your touch. That map gives her not just a greater sense of her body and senses, but also a self-awareness. Body awareness is fundamental to *self-awareness*, and both are necessary first steps to open the doors to a fuller social world where she can be aware of others around her. All this and more is conveyed through the sensitive communication of your intentional touch. With the daily repetition of QST, you deliver this 'internal guidance' as you react to her emerging feelings, fears and excitements. When you start out, you will begin by steering *for* her as her pilot, then slowly you'll steer *with* her as her co-pilot. Finally, you can sit back as her passenger and let her take the sensory controls as she begins to make sense of what were once confusing internal sensations.

As you can imagine, this becomes a very intimate, nuanced and internally focused dance that all gets communicated through your touch. You could say that the QST method is really a kind of touch language that's 'absorbed' through the skin and speaks directly to her senses, body and brain. It speaks through movement, actions and feelings. It is a message more powerful than words. You show her through what you do. You don't force or impose; you demonstrate and guide. Your touch and responsiveness speak directly to her sense of sensory overload in 'sensory-speak', the communication that an overwhelmed and frightened child understands best.

Through the language of attuned touch, you can tell your child many things. First, the consistency and predictability of your touch reassures and conveys love and safety. This happens through the affection you show, the regularity of your own movements, your own sense of calm and the responsivity to her anxious cues. Your touch also informs your child that you are keenly listening and that you will react to and respect her response when she speaks to you in that same language of 'body-speak'. Finally, attuned touch gives you a way to send a message beyond and more important than just safety – *that you can see the road ahead, that a safer and more comfortable place awaits and you know how to get her there.*

As your skill and confidence with the routine grow, you become the reliable scout in her sensory wilderness. She will come to trust that you know where you are going and that it's really okay for her to temporarily feel uncomfortable in order to get there with you. Building that trust and skill is why we focus so much on your intention while you do the routine. Your intention combines all these elements and focuses your ability to impart your more mature level of sensory organization to your child's less mature level. As we've said, QST is heart-to-heart. Now we can add that it's also sense-to-sense, body-to-body and calm-to-calm.

Co-Regulation and the Interbrain

Your child's ability to achieve self-regulation begins when you first try to find that calm and regulated state for yourself. That helps to regulate her. In turn, her cues regulate how you respond. This back-and-forth loop between the two of you is called 'co-regulation' (Ham & Tronick, 2009; Trevarthen, 1993). It is a process that can be positive, as when your child calms to your touch or soothing voice. Or it can be negative, as when your every effort to soothe your child's meltdown is met with rejection, pushing you into an exhausted and heightened stress mode where it is easy to fall into a co-escalating rather than co-regulating cycle. And, like any echo chamber, that loop can become very powerful. Co-regulation depends on a constant flow of mostly non-verbal signals that travel back and forth between you and your child. Two minds and two hearts become interconnected to the rhythm of a single heartbeat to establish one co-regulating circuit (Porges, 2015). Neuroscientists call this instantaneous bi-directional link the 'interbrain' (Schore, 2021; Shanker & Barker, 2016). Simply put, it's that innate link that you've had with your child since birth.

You can think of the interbrain as the wireless counterpart to the C-fiber highway we discussed in Chapter 3. It is a special kind of 'Bluetooth' transmission from you to your child that, while involving your touch, reaches far beyond it. It is here that everything we have discussed so far, who you are and how you impart calm and balance, is directly, immediately and 'wirelessly' transmitted to your child. It is inside this cocoon of nourishment that your child absorbs not just your knowledge and skills but, more importantly, how you sustain your connected and tender authority while still following the QST movements. Through the interbrain, she 'takes in' how you succeed or fail at taming the same dysregulations that she struggles with.

You don't have to do it perfectly every time for her to learn this skill from you! Your good intentions and best efforts are all that's needed. Perfection is not required! Remember, your child is learning not only from your results but also from your intentions and your ability to self-correct and to find a good enough way through. Each time you find that key in yourself, she will find it as well. That is all she needs to be on her way.

Speaking and Listening Through Touch

Touch constitutes the single most effective component of the complex interpersonal, nonverbal communication system . . . that underlies attachment and regulation in early life.

(Stack & Jean, 2011)

Touch as a form of communication has been with us since the dawn of time. But in our modern culture, we have mistakenly come to think of it more as an action, something we do to someone. We turn it into a simple one-way communication – that is, "I speak; you listen". We forget that it's actually an instantaneous, two-way form of communication – "As I speak, I simultaneously listen and receive a message from you". And that means when you 'speak' through touch, you're also 'listening', since you are instantly touched in turn. QST expands on this idea of touch as communication and makes it a full conversation that can inquire, inform and ultimately heal. It expands our usually limited touch vocabulary to include formal patterns of organized, intentional movements and effective responses. And it widens that language so you can talk, listen and respond in a way that goes deeper than words.

Which brings us all the way back to the first questions: "What makes QST work? What am I actually doing that makes change happen?" The short answer is that, through Louisa's unique perspective on the role of parent touch, QST gives you a means of communicating with your child in a way that she can really hear. It's a language that's primarily non-verbal because it speaks to sensory problems at the sensory level. Yet it has, as any good language has, a means to talk, listen, calm, demonstrate, teach, reassure and guide your child to a path toward growth. We are here to simply teach you the language.

Bibliography

Chapter 4

Ham, J., & Tronick, E. (2009). Relational psychophysiology: Lessons from mother – infant physiology research on dyadically expanded states of consciousness. *Psychotherapy Research*, 19(6), 619–632.
Porges, S. (2015). Making the world safe for our children: Down-regulating defence and up-regulating social engagement to 'optimize' the human experience. *Children Australia*, 40(2), 114–123.

Schore, A.N. (2021). The interpersonal neurobiology of intersubjectivity. *Frontiers in Psychology*, 12, 648616.

Shanker, S., & Barker, T. (2016). *Self-Reg: How to Help Your Child (and You) Break the Stress Cycle and Successfully Engage with Life*, Penguin Press, New York.

Stack, D., & Jean, A. (2011). Communicating through touch: Touching during parent-infant interactions. In M.J. Hertenstein, & S. Weiss (Eds.), *The Handbook of Touch: Neuroscience, Behavioral and Health Perspectives*, Springer, New York, 273–298.

Trevarthen, C. (1993). The self born in intersubjectivity: The psychology of an infant communicating. In U. Neisser (Ed.), *The Perceived Self: Ecological and Interpersonal Sources of Self-Knowledge*, Cambridge University Press, New York, 121–173.

Chapter 5

Attuned Connections and Safe Boundaries

The sensory language of QST opens new pathways of communication. Each time you adapt your touch from patting or pressing, you 'tell' your child something important. The rhythmic repetitions, the way your attuned touch 'answers' his sensory needs, the tone of your voice, the expression on your face and your own body cues all weave together to communicate a reassuring co-regulation within and through the cocoon of the interbrain connection. But there is yet another equally important communication and non-verbal guidance you convey at the same time. You might call it the structure or 'grammar' of sensory language. It involves the often automatic and subtle choices that we constantly make as we respond to our children in the moment.

Most often, these choices are well below the radar of our conscious thinking. Our child acts out, and we react automatically. When we do, we may lean more heavily toward understanding and *connecting* with our child, or we may lean more toward setting limits and *boundaries*. Both choices can be an appropriate response, but the key is to find the right *balance*. That balance, the 'sweet spot' of your relationship, blends the two essential elements necessary for your child's growing inner capacity for regulation – a feeling of being *lovingly connected* within the reassurance of *safe boundaries*.

All children need the feeling of being attuned to while cocooned *within* the experience of safe organizing boundaries. And they need to feel both from you at the same time and in the right balance. Your child's sense of *connection* comes from knowing you 'see' him, that you recognize his cues and respond to them in a predictable and attuned way. And, while feeling safe and calm, his sense of *safe boundaries* comes from knowing that you can *organize* his sensory experiences in a way that helps him make sense of the world. You could say that your child 'absorbs' through his senses how you solve a version of the same puzzle that he is wrestling with – that is, how do you manage stress and disruption while staying on task and maintaining close attunement?

QST gives you the skills to provide both *calm connection* and *safe organizing boundaries* simultaneously, blending the two through the attuned and ordered repetition of the movements each day. As you do, you fashion a 'safe container' that creates and holds these feelings of closeness and safe boundaries *for* him until he can internalize and learn to use them for himself in times of distress. Within that container, you foster and convey a fluid, dynamic balance between the two that helps your child build his own inner capacities. We believe the balance between both loving connection and safe boundaries is communicated directly through the sensory language and is key for all self-regulation. Let's look at why both key ingredients are important building blocks for growth and self-regulation.

DOI: 10.4324/9781003360421-7

Attuned Connections and Safe Boundaries

There's so much joy to be felt in slowness and softness.

Ra Avis (2021)

Connection and Slowness. Reading and skillfully responding to your child's body and emotional cues opens the doors to a deeper connection between you. And the key to attuned connection is slowing down – but a very <u>specific</u> kind of slowing down. When you slow things down in this way, you can still make a choice to do things quickly. For example, you can choose to do a quicker patting movement. But you've made that choice because it best 'fits' your child's responses at that moment, not because you rushed through just to get it done. Doing the faster movement is not about the speed, it's about taking time to observe and make a deliberate, intentional choice to respond more quickly. That's not always easy in today's fast paced world, but this kind of *focused slowness in heightened moments* is essential to how this sensory connection unfolds. When you pause and intentionally respond in a slower manner, you set yourself free from your brain's habitual and automatic ways of seeing and reacting. Your actions and perceptions become more orderly, and you become better able to see and feel your child's fast-moving responses. That gives you time to think, to feel and to respond more intentionally.

Slow is key to making a connection! It opens the sensory doors to new ways of feeling and doing. Most importantly, when you respond with this awareness, it 'tells' your child that his feelings and experiences are okay, that they don't have to be scary, that you see and respect his feelings and that he is not alone – you are there with him. With the organizing steps of QST, you provide a loving container that allows the survival alarms in his brain to turn off while instilling a sense that it is okay to relax and feel. Most importantly, it says that you are there to help him back to safety if and when those feelings spiral out of control.

Slow gets the brain's attention and creates rich new neural patterns.

Anat Baniel (2012)

Boundaries. But the road to self-regulation needs an additional, more active kind of response that organizes your child's sensory experiences and helps him make sense of them. This involves the second key ingredient to the success of the treatment: organizing boundaries. In addition to deepening your attunement, QST gives you a set of *ordered* and *predictable* steps to follow. The consistent daily repetition of the organizing touch routine gives your child's brain a sense of where his skin is, of who that person inside him is, and of where the boundaries are between himself and the outside world. Children need those boundaries to form an enduring sense of self. Children need those boundaries to feel safe. And for children who are easily tipped into survival mode, those boundaries and the sense of order they bring are especially important.

Balancing the Two

While both connection and boundaries are each equally important, neither can stand alone. The key to growth is providing them together in a balanced way. Your open responsivity nestled inside of a predictable, safe container communicates the message that it is safe to be open and connected. How you maintain your balance between attunement and the predictable safety of the organizing movements is at the heart of what QST is all about and what makes the treatment so effective.

Finding that balance in the daily routine is much like finding your balance on a bicycle. Lean too far to one side and you can focus too much on responding to your child's cues and feelings. You will make a connection and create a warm bond but may be taken off track from providing the necessary organizing boundaries and structure of the routine. Lean too far to the other side, and you can focus so intently on the movements that you miss seeing and responding to his cues of overwhelm. He is left feeling alone in his distress and you risk losing that key relatedness that makes him feel safe so his nervous system can down-regulate.

It's actually quite easy and a skill that will come naturally when you know what to look for! It is your child's body and behavioral cues that will tell you when you have gone too far to one side and need to re-calibrate the balance. Reading and responding to his sensory language is just like learning to ride a bike, you'll learn to keep the balance step-by-step each day. Like the cyclist, leaning too much in either direction can tip you over. But, just like the cyclist, you can get up and start again.

When you think about it, you are already finding that balance between connection and boundaries in almost every aspect of your life. You find that balance at work when you feel angry about an injustice yet remain professional and considerate. You find it in a dispute with your partner when you remember your feelings of love while expressing your upset. When disciplining your child, you constantly balance feelings of kindness and firmness, irritation and compassion, holding your authority and relaxing it, acting silly and being serious, and a host of other seemingly opposing demands. What we are calling balance is really just trying to find the right blend that addresses both needs, attuning to one without ignoring the other, while trying to make the best fit for what the situation calls for. Without noticing, you make hundreds of balancing judgments, continuously re-adjusting the scales of your behavior and your emotions to meet your child's needs and the needs of the moment. You maintain these balances smoothly and without thinking.

QST is about who you are as you sustain this balance between creating calm connection and maintaining safe boundaries. The essence of the daily routine is that you do both of these *at the same time* – you keep the organizing structure of the movements, held just loosely enough to simultaneously adapt your touch to your child's cues to sustain a responsive, calm connection. With QST, you'll learn quite simply to balance the two. That sets the stage for the invisible transmission that provides the basic building blocks of self-regulation. To see how this works in real life, let's take a look at two parents who initially tilt too far to one side as they learn to find their own balance.

Two Parent's Stories

Jenn: Connection Without Safe Boundaries

Jenn is the mother of two children, ages five and three. The birth of both children had been traumatic and medically complex, and she described her 5-year-old, Maggie, as a "high intensity" child from the moment she was born. Jenn came to QST looking to 'fix' Maggie's worsening problems at school (anxious behaviors, inability to control impulses, difficulty playing/sharing with others, constant tantrums with aggression toward Mom and unrelenting sleep problems). Jenn was a dedicated mother, learned the protocol quickly and had a strong desire to connect with her daughter, but within the first days and weeks of QST, she became frustrated when she couldn't get through all the steps.

It soon became clear that the treatment kept going off the rails over and over again, and in much the same way. It started out well, but when Jenn would try to do the movements in the areas where Maggie had heightened sensory issues (i.e., touch resistance on the face, head, chest, fingers and toes), Maggie would giggle and entice her mother into sweet, silly games to distract her from continuing. Jenn did not see that this was Maggie's way of distracting her from touching the painful or uncomfortable areas on her body. She responded instead by joining in a game of tickling that only heightened Maggie's over-reactive nervous system and invariably led to the whole session breaking down into a fun and hilarious romp. While this intense bubbly interaction was lovely to see, the antics derailed Jenn from completing the steps of the routine. Only able to make that all-important parent-child connection *on her child's terms*, she missed her essential co-piloting task, leaving Maggie in the driver's seat of a sensory car she was not equipped to control.

Jenn was apprehensive about touching Maggie in those areas that were painful and hypersensitive to touch. She had difficulty setting limits and boundaries, both in the treatment and at other times as well. What looked like a wonderful fun game was, from a treatment perspective, adding to the sensory overload. While a deep connection between mother and daughter was clearly evident, that form of contact, at that moment, did not provide the organization Maggie needed. Easily enticed into stopping the movements and getting drawn into the escalating play, Jenn missed the very thing Maggie's nervous system needed the most, the organizing, regulating, repetition of touch, adapted in a way that was tolerable to her. Jenn's own discomfort with authority and her feelings of guilt about being seen as 'mean' or unfair prevented her from setting these boundaries in an organized, intentional and sensitive way. Jenn's sensory 'message' to Maggie was that while it was wonderful to connect, good boundaries were unsafe, intrusive and to be avoided!

Amy: Boundaries Without Attention to Connection

Amy is the mother of a 4-year-old boy, Josh, who had "terrible sleep problems" and "extreme sensitivity to all sensory input". Even the slightest degree of touch, light, smells or sounds would send him into an intensely defensive mode, causing him to try to block out any stimulation, including touch, often ending in screaming fits and tantrums that could "go on and on". Concerned at how these behaviors were interfering with his social skills at school with teachers and peers, Josh's parents had tried a wide range of interventions, all with little or no improvement. They came to QST as a last resort.

Amy worked in a high-intensity corporate job and, as in her professional life, she learned the movements quickly and did them in a very focused and organized way. However, she was so intent upon getting through the steps as quickly and efficiently as possible that she ignored Josh's growing signals of discomfort and his tendency to resort to hitting, kicking and screaming to get away. Amy mis-read Josh's resistance and need to flee as his willfully pushing her away and did not see his cues as a heightening stress response that called for her to slow down and adapt her touch. Instead, she unwittingly intensified her efforts and pushed through the movements more quickly. When that escalated his resistance even more, Amy would give up, frustrated and exhausted, and she'd stop the treatment.

Even though her instincts told her that Josh needed "help to feel calm in his skin", Amy was, at the outset, unable to use or trust what she intuited as a parent. Instead, she persisted in following the technique without slowing down to take in either her own or Josh's cues of distress. Unlike Jenn in the previous example, Amy was able to maintain the organized steps of the treatment (boundaries), but she adhered so rigidly to the rules and structure of the movements that she missed the attuned, calming connection, leaving Josh's sensory system overwhelmed and struggling to escape.

These stories reflect common problems parents can experience. Like so many in today's culture, rushed schedules left each parent little time to attend to the cues from their children's, or even their own bodies. And their initial sense of balance in the treatment was thrown off by hidden stressors that tilted them too far away from either sensitive connection on the one hand or organized boundaries on the other. In the first example, Jenn came to see that her primary stressor was a fear that by setting good boundaries she would break the emotional link with her daughter. However, she came to understand that it was just the opposite – organized boundaries were actually the best path to quieting her nervous system and deepening that connection. In the second example, Amy's primary stressor was her personal discomfort with touch. Because she had always personally avoided it, she was tense and apprehensive about doing QST. But when each of these mothers learned to slow down and read the body cues that they had missed, they gained the confidence to respond in more effective ways and were, over time, able to follow those cues to guide their children, step-by-step to being more comfortable and regulated in their own bodies.

Communicating Balance

Without knowing it, each of these mothers tilted the balance to one side – communicating the subtle message that either attuned contact or organizing boundaries are uncomfortable and to be avoided. When the mothers were able to find a balance between the two, the sensory message they communicated told a different and more organized story, one that was tailor-made to speak directly to their child's specific regulatory needs. It conveyed an all-important message that, for their child, was easy to decipher because it spoke in the sensory language that their own body understood best. We talk to our children through our words, our actions and the subtle choices we make. But for sensory language, the communications that can speak the loudest are often the choices we don't make. Those are the ones that we tend, for our own personal reasons, to avoid or shy away from, especially when that choice may tip the balance into areas that make us uncomfortable.

When parents learn to better maintain their balance between loving connection and safe boundaries, they create the kind of *safe container* of sensations and actions that holds and organizes both themselves and their children. In fact, it is maintaining this balance that creates this container and invisibly communicates (through actions, choices and the senses) what that balance feels like and how it is achieved. You can picture this container as an enveloping bubble that you create. Nestled inside of it, your actions form secure but never rigid boundaries. It is a special adaptable container that stretches here, then holds its form firmly there as you respond to your child's body language as well as your own. It loosens rapidly when your child feels too constricted, and then gently but authoritatively re-forms when he needs a more safe containment. When your child is cradled within it, he absorbs the one skill that a sensory child needs the most – his sensory doors open wide, and he develops the capacity to 'make sense' of what his senses are telling him while maintaining the ability to stay focused on whatever task or goal he set for himself. When that happens, you've set into motion his innate capacity for self-regulation.

Bibliography

Chapter 5

Avis, Ra (2021). Interview by Kara Jillian Brown, *Poet Ra Avis Wants You to Understand that Formerly Incarcerated People are Just Like Everyone Else*, Well + Good, Mar 26, 2021. [www.wellandgood.com/ra-avis-mass-incarceration-poetry/]

Baniel, A. (2012). *Essential Two: Slow, Kids Beyond Limits: The Anat Baniel Method for Awakening the Brain and Transforming the Life of Your Child with Special Needs* (First edition), Perigee Trade, New York, NY, 77–93.

Suggested Readings

Listen – Five Simple Tools to Meet Your Everyday Parenting Challenges, by Patty Wipfler & Tosha Schore, (2016) Hand in Hand Parenting, Palo Alto, CA.

No Bad Kids: Toddler Discipline Without Shame, by Janet Lansbury, (2004) JLML Press, Los Angeles, CA.

No Drama Discipline: The Whole-Brain Way to Calm the Chaos and Nurture Your Child's Developing Mind, by Daniel Siegel, M.D. & Tina Payne Bryson, Ph.D., (2014) Bantam, New York.

Self-Reg: How to Help Your Child (and You) Break the Stress Cycle and Successfully Engage with Life, by Dr. Stuart Shanker, (2016) Penguin Random House, New York.

The Key Ingredient – You

We all know the feelings and the predictable events that follow. She collapses into a tantrum. You try everything to help. She gets angrier and loses control. Frustrated and exhausted, you want to yell and force her to comply. You may even be afraid of how angry you are. Feeling guilty you try to make amends, even abandon the rules that you normally hold. Now without those boundaries to organize her, she gets worse. You apologize, make a comforting gesture. She bats your hand away in a rage and your feelings are hurt. All your efforts have been rejected.

No matter how much we learn and how diligently we work at it, we are vulnerable to our child's next explosion and risk losing our own capacity to remain calm, focused and regulated. It's a skill that requires deep humility and a big dose of self-forgiveness. You've seen in previous chapters that how you regulate yourself is directly transmitted to your child through many channels, some we are aware of and some below our conscious awareness, both seen and unseen. These include the regularity of the QST movements, your attunement to body cues and sensory language, co-regulation and the interbrain. That's why this chapter is all about *you*. It's about how to be the best version of yourself as you do QST with your child each day, especially on those stressful days when it's hard not to take stress behaviors personally or over-react to your child's over-reactions.

It's about how one big brain, even if it is in stress mode (yours), manages to regulate and organize another smaller brain (hers) that's in an even bigger state of overload. Finding that capacity to remain calm and focused means that *who you are* as you do the treatment is as important as the QST movements themselves. The first step to finding that best version of yourself is to regulate your own feelings and emotions, *especially* when your child is in a state of overwhelm. Your child actually senses and 'takes in' who you are, and when you are calm and regulated, she 'absorbs' that from you. She also senses and takes in who you are by *how* you react to her. And, as you've seen, maintaining that balance between loving connection and safe boundaries within yourself is what makes the daily treatment so effective. This is why we feel it is important to provide you with some simple techniques to help you find that place of calm inside yourself. We start by looking at the importance of regulating your own feelings and emotions when stress clouds your ability to think clearly. To do that is easier than you might think.

DOI: 10.4324/9781003360421-8

Stress and Self-Regulation

Trying to self-regulate, especially while your child is agitated and you have too much on your plate, can be one of the most difficult tasks for any parent. You're already feeling exhausted and emotionally overwhelmed, and yet you must somehow create the ground under your own unsteady feet to provide a solid foundation for your child. It is, as the old saying goes, like trying to build an airplane while you are flying it. When you are under stress, the feeling of being overwhelmed and disorganized is much like the experience your child feels. You lose some of your capacity to think, your emotions can get the better of you and your body can feel tense and agitated. Stress, when it sets in, clouds our ability to attend to our feelings or make and follow a plan of action. It is like fog on the road or static in the TV picture. It obscures our view, disconnects us from our natural instincts and leaves us confused, uncertain and exhausted. And, as with children, stress closes our own sensory doors. It blocks access to our thinking brains and our innate parental instincts.

Stress comes to us in different forms. Some is positive, but we are focusing here on the kinds of stress that exhaust you and keep you from being your best. Some people experience it primarily as a kind of tension, tightness or pressure within their body. Muscles become tense; there is pressure in the head, chest and shoulders. Heart rate and blood pressure go up, or there is just a feeling of being 'tightly wound' with racing thoughts. Others may feel stress as primarily emotional, feeling overwhelmed, fearful, guilty, angry, anxious or sad, leaving them prone to outbursts or to spending precious energy to suppress saying or doing something they may regret. Either or both of these kinds of stressors can get in the way of finding that place of calm- connection that makes your daily treatments most effective. But most parents do find, once the static clears, that their innate good parenting skills come back quite naturally. So, let's take a look at the kinds of simple techniques and fresh ways of looking at ourselves that a busy parent can use to help find their own regulation in stressful times.

Quieting Physical Stress – Through the Language of the Body

We all know that no amount of telling ourselves to calm down works very well. That's because the best way to reduce stress is not through our mind but through our body. Actually, the most effective methods for adults to self-calm and de-stress have some surprising similarities to how you calm your child. Trying to persuade, cajole, bargain, argue with or especially force a child to calm down will either heighten their agitation or drive it further underground only to come back stronger. The same holds true when dealing with your own stress – tension will not submit to your will and, as with your child, it is best approached with softness toward yourself and supported with quiet resolve. Just as your child's sensory problems require a sensory solution, your own heightened stress also requires a body-based solution. We can best speak to our own stress in the *language* of the body.

The first step is to take a step back from the urgency of the situation. We are not suggesting something as simplistic as 'just don't get triggered'. We all react in the moment, no matter how prepared we think we are. But when you find yourself escalating, the first and most important thing to do is pause for a moment, slow down and bring your awareness directly into your body and your breath. Slowing down gets us out of automatic mode and connects us to the *feeling sense* of ourselves. Only then can we connect with others around us.

Mindsight is cultivating the ability to become aware of what is happening in your mind and brain without being overtaken by it.

Dr. Daniel Siegel (2010)

Try this simple exercise:

- Pause for a moment, and simply feel your feet flat on the floor.
- Then, without forcing it, take a slow and easy full inhale. Close your eyes for a moment as you do this and feel your breath come down into your belly. Feel your ribs, in the back and front, gently expanding.
- Now – for the most important part for purposes of finding your own calm – breathe out slowly and allow your exhale to be a little longer than your inhale.
- To lengthen your exhale, see if a sigh or quiet hum helps to extend your exhalation easily and comfortably.

Lengthening your exhale engages that part of your nervous system that is linked to the relaxation response. It slows your heartbeat, calms the body and is the first step necessary before you attempt to re-engage your thinking brain for any task ahead. Repeat this gentle inhale and exhale for 2–3 breaths and see if you don't notice your own tensions start to melt and feel a little more grounded. Relaxing into more regulated breathing will also allow you to better observe and sensitively respond to your own cues of physical tension and discomfort. As you *gently* do this breathing exercise, you will find that over time your child's breathing will start to synchronize with yours. She is not hearing your words (telling a child in fight-or-flight to take a breath almost never works), but she will take in and sense your actions. Then, wordlessly, she will often join you by deepening her own breath.

When it comes to your own physical stress, if you can't easily 'figure out' what may have caused it, don't try to explain or over-think it! Just bring your awareness to the physical sensations in your body, breathe and 'feel' into them. Sometimes, simply bringing these basic signals into our awareness, without judging ourselves or them, then giving them a name, (i.e., my stomach is in a knot, my shoulders are so tight the muscles throb) and gently breathing into them can bring a sense of release to the area. Focus on the actual sensations themselves. *What are you feeling in your body? Where are you feeling it? What is your body telling you?* Begin with a few body-focused questions to help you tune in to your body's signals in a gentle and caring way:

Where do I feel the most tension in my body? My shoulders? Neck? Back? Stomach? Hands and arms?
Am I holding my breath or breathing shallowly?
Is my heart racing? Is my chest tight?
What is the expression on my face? Is my jaw set? Is my brow furrowed?
What is the tone of my voice? Is it elevated? Is my pace of speaking rushed?

Like any good body-based exercise, the key is listening to how your own body responds. Don't force anything. Only continue with those exercises that give you a sense of calm and lower your own stress response. Your goal is the same as for your child, to get *under* the stress. We say under because we can't get over or through stress; we need to give ourselves permission to approach it through a new softer lens, one less driven by reason or logic and focused on quiet, gentle attention to the body itself.

If you still find that focusing on your body cues does not help you to calm, you have another, equally powerful tool to help you down-regulate. The QST movements you do with your child will also calm you! We've found that even the most anxious parents find solace in the rhythmic structure of the treatment. Once you've learned the movements and they become second nature to you, staying with them and doing them in their order as you focus your attention on your actions and your child's sensory cues will actually help to focus and calm you! Just as with some forms of meditating or organized-intentional movements, the 'embodied regularity' of QST over time connects parents to their own body cues and sensations. And the more you gently focus on your own sensory experience and strengthen your awareness of your own body signals, the better able you'll also be to observe, read and respond to your child's cues.

Some parents have told us that the act of calming down itself can feel stressful. That makes sense if we think of stress as the result of the huge energy expenditure it takes as we try desperately to take control when life's demands seem overwhelming. And we know that the natural tendency to race even faster just makes things worse. But when parents allow themselves to slow down and de-stress, it can feel like they are closing their eyes and taking their hands off the steering wheel of a speeding car. 'Letting go' can sometimes feel scary, but we have to trust that when we do, there is something much better ahead for ourselves and our child.

So, whether finding calm from physical stress comes from connecting to your own body's cues and trusting that it's ok to slow down or from the structure and order of the treatment itself, you will get there. Be gentle with yourself, let go of self-judgment, look at yourself through soft eyes. Do the best you can with each movement, each day.

Quieting Emotional Stress

Strong, difficult emotions and the stress that comes with them can be just as dysregulating as physical stress. While the two are deeply intertwined, your powerful emotions can be particularly de-stabilizing to you when your child erupts into an emotional storm. These storms can act like a compelling invitation and even a demand that you 'dance' with them. While we don't always have to respond to every invitation to dance, we can easily find ourselves drawn in as unwilling partners. It can happen in an instant – your child suddenly dissolves in a screaming tantrum in the check-out line and you're already late for your next appointment. You get sparked with a sudden feeling of anger in your gut. We are all susceptible. And when you add the accumulation of stress from a hard day at work to your child's meltdown, it's easy to see how an emotion can quickly hijack your body, your brain and your ability to act.

When you over-identify with your child, there are two children in the room and no parent.

Dr. Gerard Costa (2022)

As with physical stress, the first thing to do when in the grip of a strong unsettling emotion is to pause – slow down – bring your attention to your breath and focus on a long slow exhale. And just like with physical stress, locate where you are feeling the emotions in your body and use the same exercise above by gently breathing into the area. If you can't locate where the emotion sits in your body, just soften any judgment about the feelings and breathe into the emotion itself. It won't magically take the feelings away, but it often helps you to soften and down-regulate your own nervous system, just enough to get back to calm connection with yourself and then your child. That's because feeling your body-based experience can be a helpful starting point to identify and name what that feeling is.

Some of the most common emotions that we see parents struggle with include feeling *overwhelmed, anxious, defensive, irritable, enraged, guilty, afraid, ashamed* and/or *depressed*. So, once you have located where the emotion sits in your body, take a few moments to clearly name the feeling, and allow yourself to observe it – non-judgmentally. This can help to turn a vague and overwhelming experience into something more defined and understandable, and that can ultimately soften the emotion's grip. It allows you to connect to your body and your thinking brain once again. Our goal is to help you become aware of and even forgive those strong emotions and fears that naturally come up when dealing with your child's outbursts.

> *Mindsight lets us 'name and tame' the emotions we are experiencing, rather than being overwhelmed by them.*
>
> Dr. Daniel Siegel (2010)

Once you're out of the intensity of the moment and feel more connected with yourself, it can help to reflect on what sits underneath the strong emotions. We've listed some common themes and questions that help parents better understand typical emotions that pop up around the treatment. For example:

Am I too rigid or too lax around setting rules and limits?
Do I get uncomfortable showing/taking authority?
Do my child's meltdowns feel like a personal attack?
Am I too concerned about disappointing others?
Do I have a tendency to feel guilty?
Do I find touch and affection pleasurable or uncomfortable?
Do I have a tendency to retreat into my own head or rush too quickly into action?
Am I too quick or too slow to feel/show anger?
Am I comfortable or uncomfortable with feeling/showing peacefulness and serenity?

These questions and others like them help us better pinpoint and understand what we might be feeling and why. For example, if you feel *fear*, are you unduly afraid of hurting your child, feeling guilty about having 'caused' your child's sensory problems or personally uncomfortable with affectionate touch? And if you feel *pressured*, is it because you are afraid to slow down and feel discomfort with quiet and serenity or are too rigid about rules?

As you read through this list, you may find places where you recognize yourself. We've found that some of the most difficult emotions and reactions to address are the ones that touch parents most personally. While those items may be ones you need to spend more time on, we hope that just as you have softened the lens on your body cues, you will do the same with unsettling feelings. You will find that as you allow yourself to feel without judgment, you will give your own nervous system a chance to 'digest' the difficult emotion and the feeling will soften with that acceptance. All of this won't happen right away, but over time, this approach will not only lessen the emotion's grip on you but will also build the neural pathways in your own brain for self-regulation.

Now it's time to begin learning QST. We believe that with this background and understanding, you will come to see that QST is much more than just its 12 movements. When you get the feel of it, you will see that it is more like a two-part harmony where you play the rhythm and attuning accompaniment to your child's own personal melody. As you provide your child with the steadying rhythm of the QST movements in sync with your sensory attunement, you help organize her song as you harmonize her melody. You help her to develop her own, more beautiful and complex composition. You don't write the music for her. That song is her own and her personality and style can blossom.

Bibliography

Chapter 6

Costa, Gerard (2022). From personal correspondence.
Siegel, Daniel J. (2010). *Mindsight: The New Science of Personal Transformation*, Bantam Books, New York.

Suggested Readings

Everyday Blessings the Inner Work of Mindful Parenting Everyday Blessings the Inner Work of Mindful Parenting, by Jon Kabat-Zinn, Ph.D. & Mayla Kabat-Zinn, (2014) Hyperion, New York.
Parenting from the Inside Out: How a Deeper Self-Understanding Can Help You Raise Children Who Thrive, by Dan Siegel, M.D. & Mary Martzell, M.Ed., (2003) J.P. Tarcher/Putnam, New York.

Part II

Learning QST at Home

Chapter 7

Getting Started

QST is like a daily medicine for your child, a medicine that nourishes and provides a special form of 'exercise' for your child's brain and sensory nervous system. The method is simple. It works. Once you get through the initial learning curve, it only takes about 15 minutes a day. And you don't have to learn it all at the beginning. Just start with what you know, do that part of the routine every day and learn the rest as you go along. Once you begin, you'll start to see a healing and strengthening process in your child's body and feel a sense of success.

Setting Up

Before you begin, these general guidelines will help you get started in the most organized and effective way:

Pick a time that will easily become a part of your daily routine. Think about when your child would be most receptive. Bedtime often works well because the routine will help your child quiet down to sleep. Before or after school or before nap time might also work. The important thing is to set up a daily schedule that supports your ability to keep going consistently every day.

Pick a quiet, comfortable place. A favorite blanket or mat can help prompt your child to recognize that it's time for QST. Make sure it is away from any interruptions and is done where you both have the best chance of relaxing. It's equally important that you chose a place where you will comfortably be able to reach both sides of your child without feeling pain or discomfort for yourself. Some parents chose to buy a portable massage table online or use a thick blanket or pad on a sturdy table at home. Just make sure you can **protect your child from a fall if they move fast**. Above all, you must be comfortable in order to relax and sustain the treatment daily. (See Part III – Weekly Letter 2: Parent Self-Care – Finding the Right Position.)

Make sure you and your child have enough energy. Doing QST requires the energy of the person who is giving it. If you are sick, it is better to miss a day. On days when you have nothing left to give, ask another family member to take over. If no one is available, simply take the day off and wait till you are feeling better. Skip a day if your child is truly sick, but if your child is mildly ill, you might try to go ahead. You know your child best, so play it by ear.

Build a family support team. Whenever possible, encourage another family member(s) or caregiver(s) to learn QST with you, alternate giving the routine and watch the progress over the

DOI: 10.4324/9781003360421-10

year. Then, if one of you doesn't feel well, the other one can give the treatment so your child won't miss out. If both parents and/or caregivers are comfortable with the routine, they should try to give the treatment together from time to time. (See *Two Parent QST* online video – access link in Appendix H.) According to Chinese medicine, the mother and father each bring a different kind of energy to the child. Together, this makes for a wonderfully strong and balanced treatment. We know that it's not always possible to have a second person to help. So don't worry. Intention and determination will get you to your goal. We have seen plenty of parents do the program solo with good success.

Keys to Success

We've learned a lot about how parents can maximize their child's success in the 16 years we have been researching the QST autism protocol. Here are the important lessons to guide your way:

1. **Attune your touch to your child's body language.** This is the *most important* part of QST! Your child's responses and body cues will guide which touch technique you use – either quicker patting or slower, deeper pressing. It is so important that we've devoted an entire chapter (Chapter 9) to providing you a detailed list of what cues to watch for, what the specific meaning is for each cue and how to adapt your touch so your child can benefit the most.

2. **Be consistent.** Your daily consistency is the key to real improvement. So, in the beginning you'll need trust and 'stick-to-it-ness'. Our most recent three-year research study for children with autism showed that children who receive the QST routine 5–7 days a week showed greater improvements in the first half of the year than those who received less frequency. And those improvements continued to grow through the end of the year. Some children saw improvements quickly, while others made smaller improvements more slowly. A good rule of thumb to keep in mind is that the longer your child has had a condition, the longer the improvements may take. But improvements will come!

3. **Be patient and calm.** Your child learns calm from your own calm! We don't just teach you a touch technique, we also provide a wealth of knowledge and tools to help you find your own sense of calm that you automatically give to your child. When you first begin, it may take longer for your child to move from an agitated fight-flight-or-freeze mode into a relax-relate-receptive mode. And once there, she may not stay for very long. Consistent change will take some time. But with your calm, skilled and intentional touch, repeated day after day, you will help her shift more easily into her own relax-relate mode and stay there for longer and longer periods of time.

   Your touch communicates your emotions, so don't begin if you are very upset or angry. However, you may also find that your own upsets melt away as you do the treatment. Many parents find that giving QST leaves them feeling more relaxed afterwards too. Remember, touch is a two-way street, and the person giving the treatment gets the same benefits, often feeling just as relaxed as the one receiving.

4. **Don't skip the tough spots.** Very few children lay perfectly still to start, much less let you make it through all 12 steps. They may even refuse to participate. Children can

become agitated, distractingly playful or even refuse a parent's touch altogether at the outset. This is often the hardest part for parents because a parent's natural response in the face of pain and agitation is to back away or give up. Other parents get anxious and caught up in their child's efforts to provoke, distract or lead them off-track. Sometimes, parents even want to skip a whole movement because their child doesn't like it. These are all natural responses!

But the uncomfortable spots are the areas of the body that need the most help and are often keys to the biggest positive changes. When your child's agitation causes you to stop touching uncomfortable areas, *you may miss the exact areas that need your help the most*. The goal is to stay relaxed in your own body and find the way to adapt your touch so that your child can tolerate the contact. Only then can you both 'work through' those difficult spots until they become more comfortable and receptive to your touch. (Chapter 9 will give you tips on how to do this.) In time, her signs of comfort and discomfort will show you where the roadblocks are, and how best to attune your touch to work through the problems, not avoid them.

5. **Get help if you need it.** Even the most persistent of parents sometimes need extra help. Our appendix section at the back of the book offers links to find personalized help with a Certified QST Trainer in your area or through online help [Appendix D]. You'll also find guidelines to help you create your own parent support group so you don't have to work alone [Appendix E]. These and other resources will help you get through the rough spots and find others in your area to support you on your journey.

Setting Goals

When we start out on a journey, goals give us a clear long-term picture of where we want to go, motivating us along the way and allowing us to have a sense of confidence as we look back to see what progress we have made. So, let's begin this journey by picking three changes or improvements you most want to see from QST for your child. We want you to start out with your own goals, but if you feel stuck, examples of what parents often pick are things like: fewer tantrums, less aggression, better attention and improved social skills. Now choose your own personal goals and list them below:

1.
2.
3.

In Part III of this book, we offer a year of short weekly letters to support your progress. You will have the opportunity in Weekly Letter 28 – *Checking in on your goals* to list new goals and review those you just made above so that you can look back and see what you and your child have accomplished.

Measuring Progress

You are putting a lot of time and energy into giving your child the daily QST routine, so it is helpful to measure and have an accurate picture of your progress. We've found that it's easy for busy parents to miss the little day-to-day improvements that add up to big improvements over time. It's very common for parents to see their child's symptoms *today* as being the 'new normal' and easily forget that their symptoms were more intense weeks or months ago. So, to help track your progress, we've provided two simple checklists and a progress chart. The first checklist and the chart measure your child's progress. The second checklist measures your own.

Measuring Your *Child's* Progress

Sense and Self-Regulation Checklist

We include two ways to measure your child's progress beginning with the 'start date' *Sense and Self-Regulation Checklist* (page 60–61) which provides an extensive checklist of symptoms and behaviors commonly found in children with sensory and regulation difficulties. Completing this checklist gives you a baseline picture of your child's sensory and self-regulation capabilities before starting QST. It will also help you focus on what areas may need special attention. This checklist focuses on specific areas such as touch/pain sensitivity, each of the other senses, self-soothing behaviors, troublesome behaviors and various regulatory items. This scale is adapted from the measures used in all of our autism research studies and it is also used by our Certified QST Trainers to measure progress and advise parents where to focus the work and how long to continue the intervention. The goal is to see consistent improvement in the scores. We will provide this same evaluation at mid-year and year-end points so you can easily mark your progress.

QST Progress Chart

The *Sense and Self-Regulation Checklist* provides you with a very comprehensive measure of your child's sensory and regulation strengths and difficulties. But a picture is still worth a thousand words, so we also created a simple do-it-yourself chart that is quick to fill out and will provide you with a bird's-eye view of your child's progress in key areas of regulation. To see how this works, take a look at Figure 7.1 (next page). You'll see seven diagonally labeled columns that correspond to the most common self-regulatory areas. Two blank slots are provided at the far right so you can fill in other important behaviors or observations you'd also like to track. Simply circle the number in the column that corresponds to your overall sense of your child's current capacities *on average* in each column. A score of 10 is very positive with no difficulties, and a 1 indicates that area is most problematic. For example, if your child often has numerous consistent tantrums, you might circle a 3 under Tantrums, or even a 1 if they tend to be prolonged and frequent. On the other hand, if your child generally sleeps well, you may rate Sleep an 8, 9 or even a 10. Just use your best judgment when choosing a number that best reflects your child's overall abilities or difficulties in that area, and don't forget to include one or two additional items if you have specific concerns that you'd like to follow (for example, potty training or picky eating). Once you have rated all the areas, draw a line connecting the circles to create a quick, 'low-tech', do-it-yourself chart of your child's current sensory and self-regulation 'picture'.

QST Progress Chart

Sleep	Digestion Elimination	Focus Attention	Self Regulation	Social Connection	Tantrums Aggression	Touch Sensitivity	/	/
10	10	10	10	10	10	10	10	10
9	9	9	9	9	9	9	9	9
8	8	8	8	8	8	8	8	8
7	7	7	7	7	7	7	7	7
6	6	6	6	6	6	6	6	6
5	5	5	5	5	5	5	5	5
4	4	4	4	4	4	4	4	4
3	3	3	3	3	3	3	3	3
2	2	2	2	2	2	2	2	2
1	1	1	1	1	1	1	1	1

Self-Regulation Milestones

Figure 7.1 **QST Progress Chart – Start Date** – circle the number in each column that reflects your child. '10' is very positive/no difficulty, and '1' is most difficult. Then connect the circles with a line to complete the sensory and self-regulation 'picture'.

Measuring *Your* Progress

Parenting Stress Index

Another way to measure progress is to track the changes in *your* own stress level over time. It's easy to forget the impact that stress can have on us, especially when our child can't accept even our most caring efforts to help. Remember, the goal is not only to calm your child but to reduce your own stress as well! We fully expect that the routine will leave you feeling more relaxed and centered over time and that your own stress reactions will lessen. To help you measure your own progress, we have provided the 'start date' *Parenting Stress Index* (page 62). It is short and easy to complete and, taken at the start date, will give you a baseline from which to track your improving ability to handle the common stresses involved in parenting a child with sensory difficulties.

Now, Please Turn to the Next Pages and Complete the 'Start Date' Sense and Self-Regulation Checklist and the Parent Stress Index

You can complete the *Sense and Self-Regulation Checklist* and the *Parent Stress Index* right in the book, or they can be downloaded [see Appendix H, page 221] and printed out so you can include them as valuable information for your child's medical or early intervention team. You will find another set of these checklists to complete at six months, in the Part III – Weekly Letter 27 for the mid-year check-in, and again in Weekly Letter 51 for your year-end evaluation.

Sense and Self-Regulation Checklist

Name of child: _____   **Start Date:** _____

Please circle the response for each item that most accurately describes your child.

1. TACTILE = ORAL & TACTILE	Often	Sometimes	Rarely	Never
• Does not cry tears when hurt	3	2	1	0
• Doesn't notice if the diaper is wet or dirty	3	2	1	0
• Face washing is difficult	3	2	1	0
• Haircuts are difficult	3	2	1	0
• Refuses to wear a hat	3	2	1	0
• Prefers to wear a hat	3	2	1	0
• Cutting fingernails is difficult	3	2	1	0
• Prefers to wear one or two gloves	3	2	1	0
• Avoids wearing gloves	3	2	1	0
• Cutting toenails is difficult	3	2	1	0
• Will only wear certain footwear (e.g. loose shoes, no socks)	3	2	1	0
• Prefers to wear the same clothes day after day	3	2	1	0
• Will only wear certain clothes (e.g. no elastic, not tight, no tags, long or short sleeves)	3	2	1	0
• Cries tears when falls, scrapes skin, or gets hurt (Scale is reversed on purpose)	0	1	2	3
• Head bangs on a hard surface	3	2	1	0
• Head bangs on a soft surface	3	2	1	0
• Avoids foods with certain textures	3	2	1	0
• Tooth brushing is difficult	3	2	1	0
• Mouths or chews objects	3	2	1	0
Self-regulation – Orientation/Attention/Self-soothing/Sleep	**Often**	**Sometimes**	**Rarely**	**Never**
• Has to be prompted to make eye contact when spoken to	3	2	1	0
• Seems not to notice when spoken to in a normal voice	3	2	1	0
• Does not respond to his/her name	3	2	1	0
• Does not notice or react when tapped on the back	3	2	1	0
• Does not roll over onto the back when asked	3	2	1	0
• Stares off into space	3	2	1	0
• Seems unaware when others are hurt	3	2	1	0
• Has difficulty calming him/herself when upset	3	2	1	0
• Gets upset or tantrums when asked to make a transition	3	2	1	0
• Has difficulty falling asleep at bedtime	3	2	1	0
• Has difficulty falling back asleep when awakens during the night	3	2	1	0
• Awakens very early and stays awake	3	2	1	0
• Has difficulty awakening in morning	3	2	1	0
• Makes little jokes (*Answer only if your child has language.*) (Scale is reversed on purpose)	0	1	2	3
SubTotal-pg 1: _____ [Sum of all columns]	☐	☐	☐	☐

Please circle the response for each item that most accurately describes your child.

2. SENSORY = VISION	Often	Sometimes	Rarely	Never
• Looks at objects out of sides of eyes	3	2	1	0
• Is bothered by certain lights	3	2	1	0
Self-regulation – Behavior: Irritability, Aggression, Self-injurious	Often	Sometimes	Rarely	Never
• Tantrums or meltdowns	3	2	1	0
(Tantrums last_____minutes, and occur_____times/day)				
• Cries easily when frustrated	3	2	1	0
• Hits or kicks others	3	2	1	0
• Scratches or pulls other's hair	3	2	1	0
• Bites others	3	2	1	0
• Throws things at others	3	2	1	0
• Pulls own hair (Where on the head?)	3	2	1	0
• Bites self (Which part of the body e.g. left thumb?)	3	2	1	0
• Hits self (Which part of the body?)_____	3	2	1	0
• Gets aggressive or 'hyper' with exposure to certain smells	3	2	1	0
3. SENSORY = HEARING	Often	Sometimes	Rarely	Never
• Reacts poorly to certain everyday noises	3	2	1	0
• Covers ears with certain sounds	3	2	1	0
• Reacts strongly when others cry loudly or scream	3	2	1	0
• Is startled by sudden noises	3	2	1	0
Self-regulation – Toilet training	Often	Sometimes	Rarely	Never
• Is dry at night (scale is reversed on purpose)	0	1	2	3
• Diaper is wet in the morning	3	2	1	0
• Wears a diaper during the day	3	2	1	0
• Is toilet trained (scale is reversed on purpose)	0	1	2	3
4. SENSORY = SMELL	Often	Sometimes	Rarely	Never
• Gags with certain smells	3	2	1	0
Self-regulation – Digestion	Often	Sometimes	Rarely	Never
• Will only eat familiar foods	3	2	1	0
• Does not seem to be interested in food	3	2	1	0
• Eats very few foods (five to ten items)	3	2	1	0
• Bowels are loose	3	2	1	0
• Bowel movements ("poops") are frequent (more than 3 per day)	3	2	1	0
• Requires regular use of laxative to avoid constipation	3	2	1	0
• Bowel movement ("poop") is hard and dry	3	2	1	0
• Has a bowel movement every other day	3	2	1	0
• Has a bowel movement twice a week	3	2	1	0
• Has a bowel movement once a week	3	2	1	0
• Bowel movements are often green	3	2	1	0

SubTotal pg 1: _____   SubTotal pg 2: _____   Total_____

Parent Stress Index

Name of child: _____   **Start Date:** _____

Please rate the following aspects of your child's <u>health according to how much stress it causes you and/or your family</u> by placing an X in the box that best describes your situation.	Stress Ratings				
	Not stressful	Sometimes creates stress	Often creates stress	Very stressful on a daily basis	So stressful sometimes we feel we can't cope
Your child's social development	0	1	2	3	5
Your child's ability to communicate	0	1	2	3	5
Tantrums/meltdowns	0	1	2	3	5
Aggressive behavior (siblings, peers)	0	1	2	3	5
Self-injurious behavior	0	1	2	3	5
Difficulty making transitions from one activity to another	0	1	2	3	5
Sleep problems	0	1	2	3	5
Your child's diet	0	1	2	3	5
Bowel problems (diarrhea, constipation)	0	1	2	3	5
Potty training	0	1	2	3	5
Not feeling close to your child	0	1	2	3	5
Concern for the future of your child being accepted by others	0	1	2	3	5
Concern for the future of your child living independently	0	1	2	3	5
Subtotal					
Total					

Chapter 8

Qigong Sensory Treatment
Step-by-Step Instructions

My husband and I do Qigong for our son – no one can do it better than we can.

Mother of a 4-year-old

QST is an *attuned* treatment. That means that *how* you adjust your touch to make it most comfortable for your child is just as important as the 12 specialized movements you will learn here. The good news is that you know instinctively how to attune your touch to your child. You have been doing it since he was born! You know exactly how hard and how fast to pat your baby's back so that he burps, how tight to lace your toddler's shoes so that there is not too much pressure and how hard to squeeze when you give him a big hug. You might not realize *how* you know these things; it is a combination of being sensitive to your child's little sounds of pleasure or discomfort and of being aware of his smiles, grimaces and body language. You will use this same intuitive knowledge as you learn the touch techniques and hold the right intentions in your thoughts as you do the movements.

Two QST Touch Techniques: Patting and Pressing

With QST, you will be using two types of touch – *patting* and *pressing*. Watching the online instructional videos will give you a good sense of how to do both types of touch, but practicing with someone other than your child to begin will help you understand how to use an appropriate weight and speed. The **shape of your hand** is important during patting and pressing for two reasons: it ensures a more comfortable touch, and it better transmits your energy. If you think about your hand and how you use it to interact with others, you'll realize that your palm is a point of *connection* with other people. We greet people by pressing palms in a handshake. We hold hands to communicate love. So, in the QST movements, whether patting or pressing, be sure to always use a *soft and relaxed* hand to communicate these feelings.

Patting and pressing are each used for a different purpose. For most of the movements, you will be using the slower pressing movements because pressing calms a hyperactive nervous system and helps your child to tolerate touch. But there are times when patting is needed. This is especially true for some children who are on the under-sensitive side and prefer quicker patting. However, every child will at times need both: **pressing** to calm and **patting** to help foster awareness of the skin and open up energy blocks. To make your child comfortable, you may need to switch from patting to pressing several times. You can't go wrong if you let your child's body cues and instinctive preferences guide your choice.

DOI: 10.4324/9781003360421-11

Pressing Movements are Slower and Deeper

Use the entire surface of your hand, letting your relaxed palm and fingers mold to the shape of the body part you are pressing into. Pressure is firm but gentle and intentional. Keep a steady rate of about **60 beats per minute** (about one press per second), the speed of the resting heartbeat. If your child is hyperactive, you will need to use pressing for most of the movements. Pressing allows you to bring the calming rhythm of your hands to help regulate the immature and over-active sensory nervous system and to help your child tolerate and integrate more sensory input.

Patting Movements are Quicker and Lighter Than Pressing

When you pat, cup your hands slightly so you aren't using a flat hand on your child. Cupping also creates a little air space in the palm that is filled with your qi-energy. When working on your child, keep your fingers relaxed and use more of your entire cupped hand to mold to your child's body. The purpose of the pats is to activate and move the energy and circulation under the skin without it feeling hard or hurtful. To move that energy, there needs to be some weight in your pats. They must be firm, intentional and similar to the weight you might use to burp a baby where your intention is to free a gas bubble. When patting other parts of the body such as the ears or neck, your hand sometimes needs to be shaped a little differently. Here, you would use less of your palms. Around the ears and the back of the neck you'll use the flats of your fingertips (avoid fingernails). On the sides of the neck use the flats of your fingers. Use whichever helps you cover the different parts of your child's body most comfortably.

Helpful Hints for Best Results

In the following pages, instructions for each of the 12 QST movements include body diagrams that instruct you exactly where to do the movements. Here are some important things to remember to make your treatment most effective:

- **Follow the dotted lines.** When reading the diagrams, the dotted lines follow the acupressure points and channels. The movements always start on acupressure points and follow acupressure channels, which are represented by the dotted lines on the charts. These points and channels are the *doors to your child's energy* and become powerfully effective when you activate them in the right way. But you need to follow them exactly. If your downward movements are **next to** but **not on** them, you will have missed that open door.

- **Always move down the body.** Qigong movements always move downwards from the head toward the hands and feet. Never do the movements up the body. The goal is to always move the energy down toward the fingers or feet. Going in the wrong direction could give your child a headache and will interfere with his ability to relax.

- **Repetitions.** The instructions for each movement show a minimum number of times you should do each one. All are repeated at least 3x unless otherwise noted. As you become more skilled, you will find yourself repeating the movements many more times or spending more time on one body area or another, depending on how your child is responding and what he needs that day. Typically, the whole set might take 10–15 minutes, but in the beginning or on some days it may take twice that long.

- **Parent intention.** As you read the instructions for the 12 QST movements that follow, you'll notice that we've included a short 'parent intention' section in each one. These are there to help you focus on a specific goal for the outcome of each movement, and holding that intention in your mind as you do the movement will enhance your effectiveness. When you imagine intention, think of teaching your child to ride a bike. Your overall intention is that he learn to ride. To get there, you don't let yourself get too frustrated because you know he needs your patience and that it will take him some time. This knowledge helps you stay right there to guide him while understanding that he is going to learn at his own pace.

  Using your intention to work with your child's energy is just the same. You can't force your will, but your intention can guide your hands to do each movement in a way that supports your child's sense of safety as he goes through the bumps of learning something new. This, together with what you are learning and your understanding of your child, will help you decide when to continue on and when you've made enough progress for the day. So as you do these 12 Qigong movements, keep in mind what your intention is for each of them. It may be to relax your child, strengthen different areas, activate self-soothing and self-regulation, open up circulation or to provide a balanced whole-body input to your child's brain. Keeping your focused intention at the front of your mind will make your treatment even more effective.

- **Find your calm.** Before you begin QST each day, pause at your child's side and take a moment to slow down to find that place of calm inside yourself. It's not always easy in our rushed lives, but taking a moment to set your intention will help to take you there. Feel your feet on the floor and focus on a slow deep exhale. Allow your shoulders to relax. Allow your hands to relax. Then rub your hands together several times as you focus on the warmth of the loving energy in your hands. Another slow exhale and you are ready to begin.

- **Know what to watch for.** We also include a very important section on what to watch and/ or listen for in each movement. It draws your attention to a number of your child's easy-to-overlook but very important responses or actions, along with the specific meaning of each one. Learning how to identify and effectively respond to each these body and behavioral cues is such an important part of QST that we've devoted a whole chapter to it (Chapter 9). Your attunement to these cues is what gives you the vocabulary for your new 'sensory language'. Knowing what to watch for and how to respond will become one of the most fascinating, rewarding and effective parts of QST.

- **Learn the 12 movements well.** Before you begin, read this book, watch the online instructional videos and practice with a partner. There are 12 specific movements that are done in a particular order and follow a specific pattern of points and channels. It's important that you learn these well. It will help to make a copy of the *QST Sensory Movement Chart* in Appendix A (page 204) [or see Appendix H, page 221, to access downloadable copy] and have it next to you or taped on the wall where it is easy to see. It will take a while to learn it by heart but soon it will become second nature.

Please view the online videos before doing the movements.
[See Appendix H (page 221) to access videos]

The Movements

1 – Making a Connection

[Arms to hands]

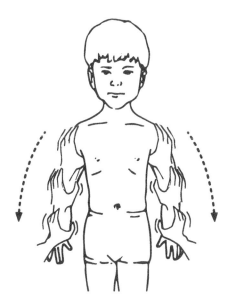

3–6x until child relaxes

Child position: Lying on the back, face-up, arms out to the sides.

Parent intention: To establish a reassuring and respectful connection with your child.

The movement: Using slow deep pressure, starting from the shoulders, gently but firmly squeeze down his arms to his hands. Repeat this downward movement several times, always starting from the shoulders down (never upward), until his arms and hands become completely relaxed. If his hands are closed into little fists, gently open them and hold them open with slow, deep pressure. Keep a rhythm of about 60 beats a minute (the resting human heart rate). At the beginning, you may need to do this more than 6 times until his arms and hands are completely relaxed.

Watch for: Big jumping movements of his arms and legs. These won't last long and are a sign that the brain is connecting pathways that coordinate the arm and leg movements. Keep going until these movements have stopped and the arms are relaxed. When they stop, your intentions will turn from working on coordination of big muscle movements to working more on fine motor awareness and communication. Look for eye contact and a smile. Your return smile will complete the connection.

Listen for: If your child speaks, be sure and respond but keep going with the routine! Your response is just as important as doing the movements correctly.

What the movement does: It brings to the brain a greater awareness of his arms and hands, increases blood circulation, opens up the channels for non-verbal communication and activates the brain pathways needed for fine motor development.

Over time: Your child will come to relax immediately, and you will both settle into the flow of the routine. Wait for your child to initiate communication and be sure to slow down and match his relaxed pace.

Signs of progress: Look for your child to show better awareness of his arms and hands and demonstrate new motor skills. He will begin to understand that this is his special time with you and develop an ease and comfort with telling you things (or vocalizing, if without language).

Optional Movement – Before Movement 2

Up – Up – Up

A QST technique for social connection

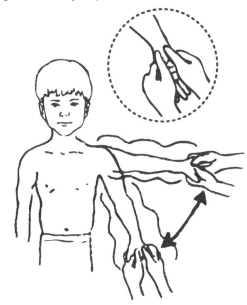

Use this movement if your child:

- Needs help opening up to social interactions
- Needs help sustaining eye contact and attention

This technique is especially useful for children who need help to comfortably engage in social interactions with peers. The movement is designed to help coordinate basic brain reflexes and engage the relax-relate mode that makes social engagement possible. Your attuned touch, along with your calm, fun and playful voice and your inviting facial expression, sets the stage and attracts face-to-face connection. The goal, over time, is to comfortably sustain that attention and relaxed social connection.

Child position: Lying on the back, face-up.

Parent intention: The goal is to attract relaxed face-to-face connection in a warm and playful way. Once you have made that eye contact and connection, your intention is to sustain your child's attention as long as he is receptive and comfortable.

The movement: Standing at your child's side, look at his face and hold his hand in both of yours. Grasp your child's hand with your two thumbs on the top of his hand at the wrist. The rest of your hand and fingers should fold around your child's hand naturally and comfortably. Your child will feel his hand is securely held when your grasp includes the palm and wrist.

Pull gently to extend your child's arm until it is fully and comfortably lengthened in a straight line from the fingers to the shoulder. You don't want the elbow to be bent.

Important Note: *be sure the wrist is in neutral, not bent up or down. It is supported in your grasp so that it remains straight and stable as you do the wave-like bouncing movement.*

If the wrist bends, it will also close off the flow of energy up to the chest. Fully extending your child's arm with enough tension allows the inflow of energy in each wave to reach and activate the chest, while at the same time allowing outflow of energy straight down the arm and out the fingers.

Start with the arm down by the side. Keeping it extended, sweep the arm upward with a bouncing wave-like motion, moving up in an arc until the arm is level with the shoulder. Pause briefly, then take the arm back down to the side with the same bouncing movement. (Think of making angel wings in the snow, one arm at a time.) Do this with a gentle, playful attitude, looking at your child's face and saying, for example, "up, up, up, up, up" as you move the arm up, and "down, down, down, down, down" as you move the arm back down.

Note: *Accentuate the "up, up, up" and "down, down, down" with a playful, sing-song quality to your voice and a fun, open expression on your face.* This is a joyful, fun and engaging movement. Please refer to online videos if you need a visual picture of how this all comes together [see link in Appendix H, page 221].

Watch for:

- *If the shoulder is tense and lifts*, use the cupped palm of your hand to do several quick patting movements across the top of the shoulder to help relax it back down.
- *If it's uncomfortable to move the arm all the way to shoulder height*, go just as far up as he comfortably allows and over time extend the range of motion as his comfort level increases.
- *Keep the extended arm in line with the side of the body* when doing the movement up and down. The chest will not be activated if you extend the arm in front of the body.
- *If your child doesn't look at you*, don't force eye contact! Just gently keep trying through your inviting facial expression and playful, sing-song voice. Direct gaze, which is very stimulating to the nervous system, doesn't always happen in the first week.

What it does: The movement sends a wave of energy into the chest to open the child's heart center, which in Chinese medicine is called the middle 'dantian' or energy center. This is the center of feelings and the desire to connect with others. The movement also coordinates the basic brain reflexes needed for your child to open up socially – the ability to face a person, comfortably make eye contact and tune the ear to the person's voice.

Signs of progress:

- Your child will make *sustained eye contact* and *connection* with you for longer periods. Over time, as he is more comfortable, he will naturally start to make those connections to other people, too.
- *A smile* says that you've had success, and that the movement is coordinating the basic brain reflexes needed for social interaction.

- *A yawn or rubbing the eyes* shows that you are activating the self-soothing capacity in his chest. Continue the movement gently a few more times.
- *If lips and tongue start moving*, then energy has flowed through the chest up to the brain and is activating the area for speech. You should continue this movement for as long as five minutes or until the lips and tongue stop moving.
- *If legs start kicking*, the energy is flowing from the chest down the legs, and he is integrating his arms with his legs. The energy flow from this movement goes into the chest and up to the face. Sometimes, it also goes down the legs. This is not kicking in a fight-or-flight way; there is much more energy to his reaction and it is often more organized. Go slower and continue the movement until his legs stop kicking.
- *As your child's comfort with social connections grow*, you may find that he no longer wants this movement and you can spend more time pressing down the arms in Movement 1.

2 – Relax Chest

[Down the chest]

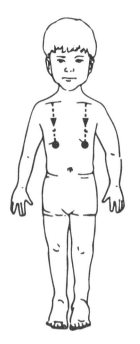

Follow dotted line, always moving downward from just under the middle of collar bone to the bottom of the ribcage.

3–6x until child relaxes

Child position: Lying on the back, face-up.

Parent intention: Relaxing the chest and activating your child's ability to self-soothe.

The movement: With both hands resting naturally on the chest, starting just under the middle of the collarbone, use the palms to press down the chest. Follow the dotted lines in the diagram above, beginning just under the collarbone to the bottom edge of the ribcage. Keep a rhythm of about 60 beats a minute (the relaxed human heart rate). Rhythmically repeat this downward movement several times, from collarbone to the bottom of the ribs.

- You are pressing about as deeply as a big hug or a deep breath. How deep you press depends on the size of your child. For the average 4-year-old, you can press down about ½ inch. It should be comfortable and very soothing.
- You may need to do this 10 or more times until his chest and breathing become relaxed.

If your child should begin to coordinate his breathing with your movements, work with him on that but do not *focus* on his breathing. In time, he should become unaware of his breathing. This is best, as it is a sign he is relaxed. If he has had hospitalizations or surgical procedures in the past, there will be areas of the chest that feel tighter than others. Do not be afraid to repeat several slow, gentle pulses on the tight areas. Stay well within your child's comfort zone. Over time, these areas will also relax.

Watch/listen for: Your child may yawn, sigh, reach up and rub his eyes or put an arm over his eyes to cover them. These are all signs that you are activating and reinforcing the self-soothing mechanisms in the autonomic nervous system. They indicate that your child's brain has switched on the self-soothing response and show that your movements are working. Each time you help your child experience this self-soothing response, he becomes better able to call on it for himself when he is stressed or overwhelmed. If your child puts his hands on yours during this movement, it's a positive sign that you are giving him just what he needs; continue the movement until he moves his hands away. This shows you are filling up his chest with calming energy and he is helping you.

After you have done this movement a number of times, it may lead to feelings and emotions coming to the surface for your child – an emotional release. (This can be especially true if your child has gone through major hospitalizations, injuries or emotional losses.) Your child's chin begins to quiver, his eyes well up with tears and he may cry. To help stay calm, take a relaxed breath and focus on a slow exhale, maintain soft eye contact and most importantly, keep going until the emotions have passed. Your touch is allowing old emotions to come to the surface and be released. Just think of it as an 'emotional bubble' that rises and pops. Your comforting touch allows it to pass, and your child will be calmer and sleep better. A gentle reassuring voice repeating, "You're ok", is most helpful at these times.

Note: Your intention behind these words is to reassure him that you are there, to make him safe and to show that it is okay to feel and express those feelings.

What it does: Your movements open up the energy and circulation to the chest. They stimulate the self-soothing response in the brain. This may also lead to emotional release if there has been some kind of trauma.

Over time, signs of progress: This movement will help you to reach an important goal – that your child achieves his self-soothing milestone. When this occurs, tantrums will be much shorter and less intense, transitions will be easier and you will see that his overall behavior becomes more flexible.

3 – Belly Circles

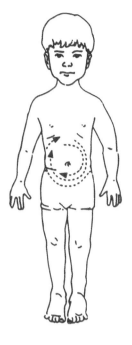

9x, 9x, 9x

(see details for direction of circles)

Child position: Lying on the back, face-up.

Parent intention: To strengthen your child's digestion so that constipation, diarrhea or reflux stop. For the child with a weak or finicky interest in food, to improve your child's appetite.

The movement: With the flat of your entire hand conforming to your child's belly, use the palm as the key place of contact to make 3 sets of 9 circles around your child's belly button. The direction of the movements will change depending on the nature of your child's elimination. For the child with:

- **Loose or normal stools** – start <u>clockwise</u>:

  9x clockwise, 9x counterclockwise, 9x clockwise.
  Clockwise movements are done more slowly and deeply.

- **Constipation** – start <u>counterclockwise</u>:

  9x counterclockwise, 9x clockwise, 9x counterclockwise.
  Counterclockwise movements are done more quickly and with a
  lighter touch.

- **When the bowels return to normal** – Loose or normal stools - Constipation - go back to starting clockwise.

Watch/listen for: Pay attention to whether your child draws his legs up or starts kicking them during this movement. If your child starts kicking, he is releasing energy from the belly down to the legs. Keep doing the movement, alternating 9x clockwise and 9x counterclockwise, until the kicking stops. End with patting or pressing down the legs until they are fully relaxed. If your child draws his legs up, switch briefly to Movement 4 – Down the Legs. Here, you will use slow deep pressure moving down his legs several times until the legs are flat. Then go back and redo the belly.

After having done the daily routine for a while, your child may release feelings and emotions stored in the belly, as sometimes also happens with the chest movement. (This may happen especially for children who have had abdominal surgery.) The released emotions usually have to do with old fears and fright. Stay calm, take a slow deep breath, be reassuring and continue doing the movement, which helps your child to release old stuck emotions. To reassure your child, you can softly say "you're OK" while you continue the movement. The intention behind your words is "it's okay to cry, it's okay to be afraid, I will keep you safe". Once your child has relaxed, move on to the next movement.

What it does: Helps clear out constipation and stop diarrhea. Stops reflux. Strengthens your child's appetite and digestive system.

Over time, signs of progress: Your child's appetite and digestion will improve. If your child was constipated, once you begin QST, you may see some black or dark green bowel movements. This is a sign that old stuck bile in the liver is moving out. It's a good sign of progress and may occur several times before the bile is all out. At that point, constipation should stop. Diarrhea and reflux will also stop, if the diet is appropriate.

4 – Down the Legs

[Front]

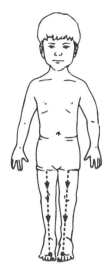

Follow dotted line, always moving downward from the top of thighs to the point on top of foot.

3–6x until child relaxes

Child position: Lying on the back, face-up.

Parent intention: To strengthen your child's legs and promote digestion.

The movement: With relaxed, cupped hands that conform to the shape of the legs, start at the top of the thighs and continue patting or pressing down the front of the legs all the way to the point on the top of the foot between the big toe and second toe. If your child is not receptive to lighter quicker patting, switch to slower deeper pressure. Make sure to *move from the top of the thigh downward* to the foot, then start again at the top of the thighs, moving always downward. (Don't make the patting motion back up toward the head.) Repeat several times.

Look/listen for: Ticklishness of the legs means that there is not enough circulation to the skin, so you will need to slow down your technique and switch to deep pressure movements. Continue this pressure downward until the legs are completely relaxed and no longer ticklish.

If your child's feet or legs are turned out too much when sitting or standing, ask your partner to gently contain them in a straight position as you do the movement more quickly and lightly with his legs straight. The quick, light patting is a strong stimulus to your child's skin and will quickly reach your child's brain and help activate the straight position of the legs. It is like you are reminding the brain to show the legs their own proper positioning.

Once your child's legs are relaxed in their proper position, change your technique to the slow pressing movements. Now you are pressing blood into the muscles so they can become stronger in their correct position. If your child's leg muscles are weak, as long as his hips are in a balanced position, this movement should be done with pressure rather than patting. Pressure will increase the circulation to the big muscles of the legs and help to build strength.

What it does: Opens up energy and circulation to the legs and feet. Improves motor development of the legs. Strongly helps the downward movement of digestion.

Over time, signs of progress: Your child's legs will get stronger. He will hold his legs in a more natural position and gross motor skills will improve. Signs of weak digestion will resolve in conjunction with changes you make to the diet. Improves the motor development of the legs. Improves digestion.

Optional – Extra Neck Clearing

[Roll over onto tummy]

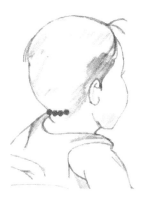

Extra Neck Clearing – Before Starting Movement 5

In preparation for Movement 5, focus attention to that part of the neck where it meets the bottom of the skull. There are many acupressure points in this area that help to relax tension in the neck and drain the sinuses.

Use this movement if:

- There is touch sensitivity on the head and neck
- Child will not lay head and body down during this movement
- Legs will not lay down flat during the movement (i.e., knees bend and heels float up)

Child Position: Lying on tummy, with face down or turned to the side.

Parent intention: To relax tense muscles in the neck and to open up channels for energy to flow from the head, down the body and to the feet.

The movement: Instead of patting with your hand, this movement is done by *tapping lightly and quickly with the flats of your fingertips* into the area shown by the dots in the figure. Be sensitive to the muscle tension under your fingertips. If your child cannot tolerate the tapping, switch to a slower pressing motion into this same area until you feel the muscles soften.

Watch/listen for: The head will lay down and the neck muscles will soften and relax.

What it does: Opens up any energy blocks in the head and allows the free flow of energy down the body to the feet in preparation for Movement 5.

5 – Down the Back – One Hand

[Down midline of back and legs]

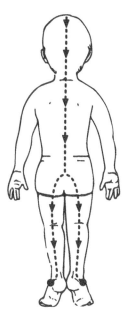

Start at center point on top of the head, moving

downward to an end at point on the outside of ankles.

3–6x until child relaxes

Child position: Lying on tummy with face down or turned to the side.

Parent intention: To open the sensory pathways between your child's brain and his back. To bring awareness of the midline of his spine and the back side of the body – from the top of the head to the outside of the feet. To relax the whole back side of the body.

The movement: Starting at the top of the head (where the infant's soft spot was), use a relaxed cupped hand, to pat *down* the body in a line that follows the midline of the head, neck and spine, until you reach the hips.

- At the hips, switch to using both hands at the same time and smoothly continue the movement down the midlines of the backs of both legs, ending at the outside of the ankles.
- If not receptive to patting, immediately switch to a slower, deeper pressing movement.
- Always move downward from the head to the heels.
- Repeat at least 3x until the body is relaxed.

Watch/listen for: The goal is for your child to lay his head down. If he doesn't lay his head down at the start, continue the movements on the top of the head until the neck relaxes and his head lays down, then continue the movement down the back. Watch for:

- *Ticklishness:* If your child shows ticklishness (giggles, cringes), slow down and switch to deeper pressure movements.
- *Arching*: If your child arches his back, keep patting (or pressing) on the spot that triggered the arching until he relaxes. Arching means he needs extra activation in that area.

- *Humming*: Listen for humming. If your child hums, it means he is joining in with your movements and that he needs you to spend extra time on that spot. Continue the movement on that spot until the humming stops.
- *Heels drifting up:* If your child's knees bend and his heels drift upwards, make several extra passes from the knee downward until his legs become relaxed and lay flat.

What it does: Opens up energy and circulation to the nerves and muscles on the back of the body and strengthens the back and the legs. Opens the senses and activates an awareness and feeling sense of the body. Helps your child let go of tension and relax into sleep. Improves your child's gross motor development.

Over time, signs of progress: Your child will fall asleep more easily and stay asleep longer. Gross motor development and muscle tone will improve.

6 – Down the Back – Two Hands

[Down sides of spine and back of legs]

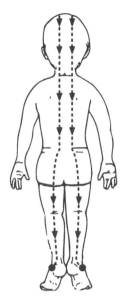

Start at the two points at the top of the head, moving downward

to an end at point on the outside of ankles.
3–6x until child relaxes

Child position: Lying on tummy, with face down or turned to the side.

Parent intention: To open the sensory pathways between your child's brain and his back and bring an awareness of the whole back side of the body, from the top of the head to the outside of the feet. To relax the whole back side of the body.

The movement: Using two hands, start from the top of the head (on either side of where the infant's soft spot was) and using either patting or, if sensitive, slower deeper pressure movement down the body. Follow the dotted lines *downward* on either side of the spine. Continue down the midline of the hips, backs of both thighs and lower legs, ending at a point on the outside of the ankles.

- Repeat at least 3x, always starting at the head and moving downward to the feet until the body is relaxed. (Always move *downward* from head to feet. Never back up toward the head).

Watch/listen for: The goal is for your child to lay his head down. Focus on the top of the head until the neck relaxes and then continue down the back. Watch for:

- *Ticklishness*: If your child shows ticklishness (giggles, cringes), slow down and switch to deeper pressure movements.
- *Arching:* If your child arches his back, keep patting (or pressing) on the spot that triggered the arching until he relaxes. The arching means he needs extra activation in that area.

- *Humming:* Listen for humming. If your child hums, it means he is joining in with your movements and that he needs you to spend extra time on that spot. Continue doing the movement on that spot until the humming stops.
- *Heels drifting up:* If your child's heels drift upwards, make several extra passes from the knee downward until his legs become relaxed and lay flat.

What it does: Opens up energy and circulation to the nerves and muscles on the back of the body and makes the muscles stronger. Helps your child let go of tension and relax into sleep. Improves gross motor development. If your child has trouble with either too much or not enough sensitivity on his skin or is slow to potty train, you can do extra repetitions of this movement. Makes toilet training easier.

Over time, signs of progress: Your child will fall asleep more easily and stay asleep longer. Gross motor development and muscle tone will improve. Toe walking will diminish. Your child will become more aware of the feeling of a wet or soiled diaper, while he also becomes more aware of his internal body signals, including his need to use the toilet. Struggles with toilet training improve. Over-sensitivity or under-sensitivity of the skin improves, and clothes feel more comfortable.

Optional – Extra Ear Clearing

[Roll over onto back]

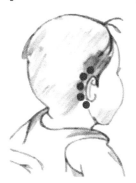

Extra Ear Clearing – Before Starting Movement 7, and/or (as Noted on Movement Chart), Before Movement 8

If the ears are sensitive to touch, it helps to give extra attention to the area around and just behind the ears. There are acupressure points in this area that help to keep the ears open, draining and comfortable.

Use this movement if:

- There is touch sensitivity in or around the ears.
- There have been repeated ear infections or trauma in the area.

Child position: Lying on back with face up or turned to the side.

Parent intention: The goal is to make touch more comfortable around the ears, reducing congestion and opening the ear.

The movement: *Using the same tapping movement you used to clear the neck, use the flats of your fingertips* to tap lightly and quickly into the area around the ear (shown by dots around the ear). Do one side, then the other.

- Here you are using a cupped hand with your fingers slightly spread, allowing the flats of your fingers to naturally make contact with all of the points in the arc around and behind the ear.
- You are not actually patting the ears with your palm. That would hurt. You are not resting your palms on the ears. Be careful to spread your fingers so that air passes between them. You don't want to be pushing air into the ear itself.
- Be sensitive to the muscle tension under your fingertips. If your child cannot tolerate the tapping, switch to a slower pressing motion. The goal is to find the touch your child can tolerate so you can continue the movement into this area until you feel the muscles soften.

Watch/listen for: The more you do this movement, the more you will become aware of the tightness or softness in the muscles that your fingers are tapping on. When you feel tightness, keep tapping on the area until you feel the muscles soften and tightness relax.

What it does: Opens up any energy blocks in the ears and allows the free flow of energy and circulation down the body to the hands and feet in preparation for Movement 7 and/or Movement 8. Helps to reduce ear congestion as much as possible so that your child can hear clearly. If the ears are congested, hearing will sound as if under water. Any blocks in the ears and hearing make it very difficult to learn language or pay attention.

7 – Down the Sides

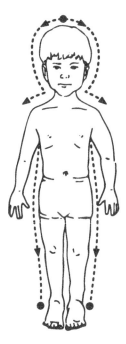

Start at the center point at the top of the head, moving downward, over the top of the shoulders.

Movement continues under the armpit – downward along the sides of the chest and body to an end at point on the outside of the ankles.

3–6x until child relaxes

Child position: Lying on his back, face-up.

Parent intention: To relax the shoulders and the sides of the body.

The movement: This movement is done with *both hands moving together down both sides of the body at the same time*.

- Starting at the top of the head (where the infant's soft spot was) and *using the flats of the fingertips* with either patting movements or, if sensitive, slower deeper pressure to move down the sides of the head, behind and around the ears.
- Just under the ear, continue to press or pat with the flats of your fingers down the sides of the neck, onto and out over the shoulders.
- Then move your hands under the armpits and continue the movement down the sides of the body. Use your relaxed, cupped hands to continue the patting or pressing movements down the sides of the body, then down the sides of the legs to the outside of the ankles.
- Repeat at least 3x until the shoulders and body is relaxed.

Watch/listen for: Ears that are no longer sensitive or painful to touch. Tension around the ears and on the shoulders softens and relaxes. Be sure to pat on the shoulders until they become loose and relaxed under your hands. If your child is ticklish on the sides of the body, switch immediately to slower, deeper pressure.

Note: If your child gets angry easily, hits, kicks or bites, this movement can be challenging at first. Take a few breaths and focus on lengthening your exhale to center and calm yourself as you continue. After a few weeks, it will get easier, and the aggression usually stops altogether. (See also Weekly Letter 33, page 175.)

What it does: Opens up energy and circulation to the nerves and muscles on the sides of the body. Relaxes the muscles around the ears and on the shoulders. Opens sensory pathways from your child's brain to the sides of the body which brings body awareness to these areas and improves motor coordination for cross-body alternating hand and leg movements. Strengthens the body's ability to eliminate toxins.

Over time, signs of progress: Improvement of motor skills. Your child is able to tolerate touch around his ears, on his neck and down the sides of the body.

8 – Ear to Hand

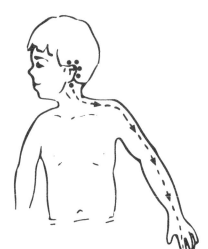

Movement starts at points around the ear.

3–6x until child relaxes

Child position: Lying on his back, face-up.

Parent intention: To relax the neck, shoulders and arms. To relax the muscles around the ears and sides of the neck.

The movement: This movement is done on one side at a time.

- Hold your child's hand in one hand. The fingers of your other hand naturally cup the ear, so they are positioned on the points just above, behind and below the ear (shown above). With the flats of your open fingertips, tap lightly and quickly into those points. Switch to slower pressing if the area is uncomfortable.
- Continue the movements with the flats of your fingers down the side of the neck.
- Smoothly switch to using the entire surface of your hand and continue the movement onto the top of the shoulder, down the top side of the arm and finish on the back of the hand that you are holding.
- Repeat the movement 3x, always starting with cupped fingertips around the ear and then moving downward over the neck, the shoulder and top of the arm to the top of the hand.

Watch/listen for: Softening and relaxation of any tension in the muscles around the ears and on the shoulders. If you find any tight or tense muscles, keep tapping or patting on those areas until they relax. Switch to slower, deeper pressure if patting is uncomfortable. If your child has had a lot of ear infections, this area is often uncomfortable in the beginning.

What it does: Opens up energy and circulation to the nerves and muscles around the ears, shoulders, arms and hands. Helps to keep your child's ears open and draining properly.

Over time, signs of progress: Less ear congestion and discomfort or sensitivity around the ears. Improvement of oral-motor sensations necessary for language.

9 – Fingers

[Down sides of fingers]

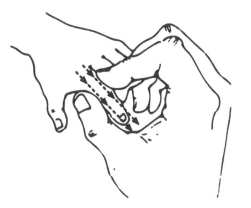

3x for each finger

Child position: Lying face-up on back.

Parent intention: To bring circulation, energy and awareness to your child's fingers. To make the fingers completely comfortable to touch. If they are uncomfortable, be ready to switch from rubbing to slower pressing.

The movement: Press down the *sides* of each finger with a pulsing pressure motion, gently stretching the finger out as you move down to the fingertip. If the fingers are uncomfortable or sensitive, switch immediately to pressing gently but firmly on both the upper and bottom surfaces of the finger. Do each finger once, then repeat a second and then third time.

- For hyper-sensitive fingers, wrap your hand around each of your child's fingers, one at a time and use a gentle, enveloping squeezing pressure.
- Don't give up on hyper-sensitive fingers. It is important developmentally to help normalize touch on the fingers.
- Once the fingers are more comfortable, the goal is to do the movement down the sides of the fingers.

Watch/listen for: Movements of your child's lips and tongue. You may see little areas move under his cheeks or under his lips as his tongue explores the inside of his mouth. If you see these movements, do not draw attention to them but continue rubbing the fingers for several minutes. This is a good sign that touch sensations are normalizing inside the mouth and lips.

What it does: Touch on the fingers stimulates the speech area of the brain and helps activate speech development. Activates fine motor development.

Over time, signs of progress: Your child's fingers will become quite comfortable to touch. Improvement of language and fine motor skills.

10 – Relax Legs

[Back of leg to heel]

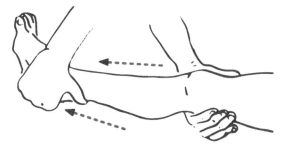

Repeat until legs relax

Child position: Lying face-up on back.

Parent intention: Settle and calm the nervous system and bring circulation down to the feet.

The movement: This movement is done one leg at a time, alternating movements from the outside/back of the leg, to the inside/back of the leg.

- To begin the movement, cup your child's heel firmly in one hand. Be sure to use a firm, grounding grip on the heel. With the other hand, start just above the back of the knee. Firmly and slowly stroke down the outside/back of the leg, from just above the knee and moving downward to the outside of the heel. When you get to the heel, let go of the hand holding the heel and firmly grasp the heel with the hand that just did the stroke.
- Now use the hand that just let go of the heel to reach up just behind the knee and stroke down from the inside/back of the leg to the inside of the ankle.
- Switch hands and continue these rhythmically alternating movements until the legs are relaxed, like 'wet spaghetti' legs.

Watch/listen for: Signs of withdrawal or discomfort with stroking. If you see these, switch immediately to deeper pressing movements down the backs of the legs, from just above the knee to the heels.

What it does: Settles your child's nervous system down and brings circulation to the feet. Relaxes your child for sleep.

Over time, signs of progress: Improved gross motor development. Falls asleep more easily.

11 – Toes

[Down sides of toes]

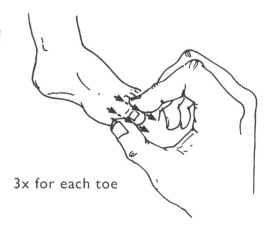

3x for each toe

Child position: Lying face-up on back.

Parent intention: To bring circulation and energy into the feet and toes and make them more comfortable to touch. This may take a while if the toes are sensitive to touch at the beginning.

The movement: Rub down the sides of each toe with a pulsing pressure (as you did with the fingers), gently stretching each toe as you move down to the tip. If your child's toes are too small for your fingers to get between them, press down the upper surface and bottom surface of the toes instead. Do each toe once, then repeat all a second and third time.

Watch/listen for: Signs of discomfort such as withdrawing the foot or ticklishness. If that happens, switch immediately to pressure on the top and bottom of the toes. If that still doesn't relieve the discomfort or ticklishness, you can guide your child's leg into a bicycle movement (this will greatly increase circulation to the feet) and then press the tops and bottoms of the toes, one by one, as you bicycle the leg down. If one toe is more sensitive than the others, it can mean it needs some extra help and you can do a little extra pressing on that toe.

What it does: Brings circulation and awareness to your child's toes. Toes and feet become more comfortable to touch.

Over time, signs of progress: Your child's toes will become quite comfortable during QST, and he will come to enjoy and relax at your touch. This will help your child with gross motor skills.

12 – Nourish and Integrate

[Rhythmic wave – feet to head]

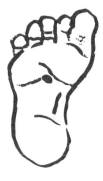

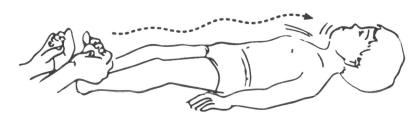

3–6x until child relaxes

Child position: Lying face-up on back.

Parent intention: To help your child integrate, through his whole body and brain, all of the organized sensory input you have given during the QST treatment.

The movement: Make sure you child's legs are straight and his face and chin are in the midline.
   Take a foot in each hand with the thumb and forefinger positioned as shown above. If the feet are initially too sensitive, use the center of your palms in place of the thumbs to press on the same point on the soles of the feet as shown above. Now, rhythmically press forward on the balls of the feet, 9 times in a slow pulsing motion. Repeat 3 sets of 9 pulses. You can quietly count out loud if that helps to keep count. Once your child relaxes into the movement, you'll be able to see his chin joining in the rocking motion, sending a pulsing wave of gentle movement up through the body at the same slow pace of 60 beats/minute that you have been using. This is a gentle rocking, slow movement of you and your child in unison.

Watch/listen for: You may see small twitching movements in your child's face, for example, lips twitching or eye lids blinking. These are signs of progress and indicate that your child's brain is making connections. Just keep silent and gently continue.

What it does: Helps the brain integrate sensory information from the whole body.

Over time, signs of progress: Over time you will see signs of overall improvement.

Rest: The Important Last Step

It is important to let your child rest once you've finished all of the movements because it enables your child's body to integrate the treatment. Once you have finished, let him lie quietly for as long as he likes. This can take a matter of seconds or can be as long as several minutes. When he is ready, he will get up on his own or go off to sleep. Follow your child's lead.

Parent Support Hands

You can see an example of what we call 'parent support hands' in the online videos where, as one person does the movements, the other person quietly places one hand on the child's chest and one on the forehead, or one hand on the chest and one on the belly. In this way, a second person can support the treatment by quietly providing a confident reassurance. In the Qigong tradition, we see this as a direct way to give energy to the child's brain, heart and gut. We have found that the feminine energy (yin) works best for the upper part – the chest and forehead, while the masculine energy (yang) is best for the lower part – the chest and belly. Using 'parent support hands' makes the treatment stronger and more nurturing. And children love it! (See also Part III – Weekly Letter 14, page 144)

Chapter 9

Reading Your Child's Body Language

Once you've learned the 12 QST movements, watching for your child's reactions and understanding how to respond to them will become one of the most fascinating and rewarding parts of the treatment. Becoming familiar with your child's unique cues and their meaning is as important as the actual QST technique for the success of your treatment. We've listed important body cues below, along with their specific meanings. It is like learning to dance together. By reading and responding to your child's cues and adapting your touch to them in the treatment, you are guiding him to learn a new and more organized way of integrating his sensory input. Over time, your organized and calming actions will slowly replace the more immature and disorganized reactions that had been all he knew.

The 'just right' touch

It is all about finding the right touch, at the right moment, for the right part of your child's body. You've already been doing this quite naturally for your child's entire life. When you found the best way to burp him or how to move his sleeping body from the car to his bed, you were adapting your touch to his response in the way you knew best.

Important Cues to Look for and What to Do

The following list includes the most common body cues and behavioral responses that are important to watch for as you do the daily QST routine. You have seen some of these before in the *Watch/listen for:* section of each of the specific movements in Chapter 8, but we list them again here, in alphabetical order for easy reference. (See also the Reading body cues – quick reference chart in Table 9.1 that follows.)

Arms and legs alternating. During Movement 7 down the sides of the body, a child will sometimes move an opposing arm and leg together (e.g., the right arm and the left leg move, or the left arm and right leg move at the same time). This is a good sign! The channels that run down the

DOI: 10.4324/9781003360421-12

side of the body are activating and you are successfully moving energy down the body. Continue doing the movement until the response stops.

Back arching. This means that you are successfully moving energy from the head down toward the feet. Repeat the movement until he relaxes or stops arching. Gently guide him with your hands to lie back down.

Belly discomfort. If your child won't lie on his belly, even if you give him helping hands to get there, he probably has a block in his belly. For belly circles in Movement 3, be sure to start with the *counterclockwise* motion, which will make him comfortable over time. In the meantime, don't force it. You can do Movements 5 and 6 with your child sitting, standing or lying on his side until he is comfortable lying on his belly.

Burping or coughing. This most commonly occurs during Movement 2. It means that energy is moving into a block in the belly. These are not literal blocks in the stomach or intestine per se; they are blocks to the channels that send energy to the digestive system so it can work properly. Stop doing Movement 2 and progress to Movement 3 on the belly, moving in a *counterclockwise* motion to relieve the block. After the block is cleared, the coughing or burping should stop. In the case of chronic constipation, it can take several weeks for the blocks in the belly to clear.

Discomfort or pain. When your child expresses discomfort, our natural instinct is to pull away and stop what we are doing. Discomfort or pain during one of the QST movements means that you've found a problem area. It is especially those areas that QST is intended to help. You just have to find the right kind of touch to address the discomfort. You might need to tap quicker and lighter, do more repetitions or switch to pressing with deeper and slower pressure until you find the touch that makes your child most comfortable. Your child's reactions will determine the correct approach. It is important to remain calm and reassure your child that "You're okay, you're okay."

Ear discomfort. Sensitivity around the ears is one of the most common problem spots and can arise from many causes, but most often from repeated ear infections or trauma to the area. Chinese medicine refers to the problem as stemming from either an 'emptiness' (lack of energy), or 'blocked' energy flow – not in the ear canal itself, but in the channels that provide energy to the area. In either case, your child will avoid patting on his ears, so try gentle rhythmic pressing *around* the ears. What you do next will depend on how he reacts to the switch to pressing. If pressing feels better and is welcomed by your child, that means the ears are empty. If he doesn't like pressing, it means his ear is blocked. Here is what to do for both:

1. **Ears empty**: If pressing around the ears feels better, you can use rhythmic pressing, along with your intention to start to 'fill' the empty area with your energy. Continue to do the slow pressing technique as you go to the next movement, 'ear to hand' (Movement 8), all the

way down the side of the neck to the back of his hand. Repeat many times until the area is fully relaxed; that is your cue that the energy has filled in.

- If you are filling the ears and your child suddenly reacts with pain, it means that the energy has percolated inwards and found a block. You should immediately change to a fast and light patting hand in order to clear the block. After a few passes, when the shoulders are again relaxed, you can try filling again. Sometimes several layers of your child's energy can clear and fill in one session. Often there is a layer of emptiness under a block where energy has not flowed for some time.

2. **Ears blocked**: If he doesn't like pressing, it means his ear is blocked and your child may refuse both patting and pressing. Most commonly the right ear is blocked, but sometimes both are. The best way to de-block the ear is for one parent to pat quickly and lightly over the ear with fingertips pointed toward the back of the head, while a second person pats quickly and lightly on the top of the shoulder until the shoulder relaxes completely. While patting the shoulder, you can intersperse several passes of patting down the arm. This moves the energy through the ear and down to the arm, so you can now do the whole of Movement 8 down to the back of the hand. See online video for Movement 8 [Appendix H]. If you don't have another family member to help, you can do the same by tapping with one hand around the ear and with your other hand patting on the top of the shoulder. It will speed up progress when you pat both simultaneously (see also Weekly Letter 17, page 149).

- Sometimes the ear will be fine one day and then not fine another day. If this happens (and your child is not sick with an ear infection), it means that you have cleared the surface layers of the ear and now have reached a deeper layer where you have found a block that needs to be cleared.

Emotional releases. Not every child will have an emotional release during QST, but we want you to be prepared so you don't get frightened. While your natural instinct may be to stop and comfort your child when you see emotions start to surface during the treatment, it is more important that you keep doing the very QST movement that triggered the reaction. Don't stop! It is your touch that is helping old emotions come to the surface and release, like an 'emotional bubble' that rises and pops. Just stay calm. Take a deep breath and slowly exhale, maintain gentle eye contact, slow the movement down and stay with it until the emotion is completely released. Your reassuring touch and voice will give a sense of calm and safety to the experience and help release the emotions that have been stored as tensions in his body. Once the emotional tension is out, he will be done with it, and you can continue with the rest of the routine as you would on any other day.

Some of the deeper emotions such as sorrow or grief may not appear until after several months, while others will commonly arise only with specific movements. For example, you may see sorrow or grief arise when doing Movement 2 on the chest. Fear, shock or even anger may bubble up when working on the belly in Movement 3. Emotions that come out like this are a sign that the area you were working on has been holding on to these emotions and that they are now opening up and healing. It's a wonderful sign that the QST is working, and it is pretty likely that you'll see some positive changes in your child's behavior following such emotional releases.

Eye rubbing. If your child raises his eyebrows, blinks his eyes or rubs them, it means you have succeeded in moving energy down from the top of the head in a downward direction. Congratulations! Stick with whatever movement you are doing. Do extra movements as necessary until the reaction stops. If you are doing Movement 1 or 2 when this happens, it means you are activating the capacity to self-soothe.

Feet sensitive or painful. It's common for a child to refuse to take his shoes and/or socks off for QST. This simply means that his feet are particularly sensitive and he's trying to protect them. The sensitivity comes from an extreme lack of circulation or energy (emptiness) in the toes, which can take several months to fill. The toes are usually the last area to 'fill up'. The goal is to do QST on bare feet, but you may have to start by pressing the toes through the shoes or socks. Encourage your child to take off their shoes and socks each time, but there is no need to fight or be forceful; if his feet are that sensitive, the skin-to-skin touch would be too much. Just press as well as you can, try to move toward softer shoes or just socks when doing this movement and stick with it. It will change. If you can't hold the feet properly for Movement 12, try resting your palms on the soles of the feet and do the rocking motion with the palm of your hands. (See also **Ticklishness**.)

Fingers ticklish or painful. If the fingers are ticklish, revert to the pressing technique on the tops and bottoms of the fingers instead of the rubbing movement down the sides. Wrap your hand around each finger, one at a time, and press it gently. Press for as long as feels good to your child. If the fingers (and it might be different for different fingers or different hands) are painful and sensitive even to pressing, try gently kneading the front of the armpit until it relaxes, press down the arm to the hand several times and then try the fingers again. Just respond to your child's reactions with pressing or light rubbing as needed (press for ticklishness, rub for pain). Over time, the ticklishness or pain will subside, and you will be able to do the movement normally.

Hand gestures. If your child puts his hands on yours during any movement, it can mean one of two things:

1. **His hands are gently placed on yours.** This means you are using just the right touch and your child needs your energy exactly there. Slow down and stay on that area. Your child will let you know when it's time to move on by moving his hand away. Here are two specific instances to look out for and how to respond:

   - **Belly**: If he puts is hands on yours during Movement 3, when you are rubbing his belly, slow down both the clockwise and the counterclockwise motions.
   - **Forehead**: Sometimes, several months into the program, a child will suddenly place the parent's hand on his forehead. This is a wonderful sign that means his brain has begun to 'fill'. If this happens, stay with it, and let your energy help to fill up his energy reserves in this area. Watch over the next few days. He will probably demonstrate a new skill or may even develop a sense of humor.

2. **His hands push yours away.** This means you need to adapt your touch or you are on a blocked area. Pat faster and lighter, but stay on the area unless you are triggering a violent fight-or-flight response. Two areas to look out for are:

- **Ear**: If you are working on the ear when you get this response, pat the ear with one hand and the top of the shoulder with the other at the same time or try patting down the arm several times starting just below the ear. Then pat around the ear again (see **Ear discomfort**).
- **Belly**: If you are rubbing on the belly in Movement 3 when your child pushes your hands away, either switch to the counterclockwise movement if you are going clockwise or make your clockwise motion faster and then pat the energy down the legs as you would if you were doing Movement 4. You might have to rub and pat, rub and pat, several times before the block clears.

Humming. If your child begins to hum during QST, it means that a block is clearing but that this area still needs your energy. This most commonly occurs when you pat down the back or on the chest. The humming signals both your child's pleasure and his relief in opening up. Humming is his contribution to that good feeling. When working on the belly, if your child starts with a low-pitched hum, do the circles slowly, staying with the same direction until the humming stops. When this area fills, enhanced vitality and health soon follow because the belly holds an important reserve of energy for the body. No matter the area, wherever the humming starts, continue patting on that spot until the humming stops. Once it stops, continue on and complete the rest of the movement. When you have finished the movement, repeat that same movement again, spending a little extra time at the same spot to see if there is more to be done there. As long as your child is humming, important things are happening.

Hyper after QST. If your child is hyper after the treatment, it means that the energy is not yet flowing down from the head. While you have most likely moved it downward during the routine, it is flaring back up and bouncing against blocks in the head, ears or neck. Find where the block is by tapping lightly until you detect where your child is sensitive. Make several light and quick passes down through the sensitive area to unblock it. The hyper behavior provides important information because it tells you that the next time you do the treatment, you should spend more time on the first six movements. Also, until you have moved the energy down from the head to the toes, you should do the treatment earlier in the day.

Jumping up during QST. If your child starts QST lying down but then suddenly jumps up, it means that you have succeeded in getting the energy to move down, but it has now encountered a block and is bouncing back. Concentrate your patting on the area that triggered the response until you can guide him to lie down again.

Leg movements. How your child's legs move during QST can tell you a great deal about what is happening in his body during the treatment. Here are some common things you may see and how to best respond.

1. **Lower legs and heels float up (when on his belly)** This means there isn't enough energy flowing down from the back to reach his heels, causing them to drift up. Do some extra strokes from the knees down until his heels can stay down.

2. **Legs kicking (when on belly or back).** Kicking when your child is on his belly is different from when his knees bend and his heels float up. Here, there is much more energy to his reaction, and it is not kicking in a fight-or-flight way. When on his back, kicking of the legs during Movement 1 as you squeeze down the arms or during the optional Up-Up-Up Movement, means that your child is integrating the connections between his arms and legs. This is a good sign! It means you've gotten the energy to flow from the chest down the legs and he is integrating his arms with his legs. Go slower and continue the movement until his legs stop kicking. Kicking when doing Movement 3 on the belly tells you that the block is clearing from the belly down the legs and that your child is helping to move it out.

3. **Legs and knees draw up toward the chest (when on back).** This most commonly happens as you do the belly circles during Movement 3. Your response depends on which direction you are rubbing when the legs come up.

   • *If rubbing counterclockwise*: During the counterclockwise part of Movement 3, there can be some discomfort if there is an energy block in the area of the belly. When this happens, your child commonly draws his legs up toward his chest. This means the energy needs to first be moved down his legs before you continue. Stop Movement 3 and pat down the tops of his legs several times (as in Movement 4*)* until his legs relax flat. Then go back to the counterclockwise motion on the belly. You might have to repeat this process several times. Start the counterclockwise motion, pat down the legs; resume the counterclockwise, pat down the legs; try the counterclockwise again, pat down the legs, etc. You'll know you've released the energy block when you can do three sets of nine circles going counterclockwise without a reaction. Unfortunately, there are many layers of energy in the belly and you might have to do the same thing again tomorrow or the next day, but look at it as a sign of progress. If the blocks are there, you want to move through all of them over time.

   • *If rubbing clockwise*: The legs coming up during the clockwise motion means that your child is trying to pool energy in his belly reserves as you send it inwards with your clockwise rubbing. This is a good sign that you are successfully helping that area to fill with good energy. Your child's legs coming up are his way of helping you.

Lips and/or tongue move during QST. What you are looking for here is puckering of the lips and/or rolling or poking of his tongue along the inside of his cheeks or mouth. These movements are reasons to celebrate, especially when you are doing Movement 9 on the fingers, which opens up your child's social abilities and makes the connection between the physical ability to speak and the speech centers in the brain. You are watching the connections happen before your eyes. Keep repeating the movement until the response stops. This can sometimes take as long as five minutes, but it is a very exciting and fruitful sign of progress.

Ribs stiff or tight. There are small muscles between the ribs which allow for flexibility of the ribcage. Sometimes, during Movement 2 on the chest, a child will have less flexibility in one specific area. This can mean there is a block in the area beneath the ribs, often in the lungs, something commonly found in children with asthma. When the blockage is in the area of the lower right rib cage, it can reflect what Chinese medicine considers a block in the liver. If on the lower left, it suggests a block in the stomach and spleen. If you suspect the lungs (right), do more of Movement 6 down the back, concentrating at chest level, always moving the energy down the body to the feet. If you are concerned about a block in the liver, stomach or spleen areas (left), begin in the counterclockwise direction when you get to Movement 3.

Ticklishness. A ticklish spot is a sign that you've hit an empty area lacking in energy or circulation. Switch immediately from patting to a slow pressing hand for that area. It might take a few days before you can switch back to patting, but stick with the slower, deeper pressing motion until the ticklishness resolves. Almost all of the movements can elicit this ticklish response. If there is a lot of emptiness in the head and neck, you'll often find more ticklishness throughout the body.

If ticklishness occurs in the toes, especially during Movement 11, shift from rubbing down the sides of the toes to a slower and deeper pressing movement on the top and bottom of each toe. If the ticklishness still persists, switching to a bicycling motion of the legs can help. Try firmly holding his heel in one hand and moving the leg in a bicycling motion while you press each toe with the other hand. Use this rhythm: bicycle the knee up and then press on the big toe as you are bicycling that same leg down. Then bicycle the knee up again and as you bicycle the leg down this time, press on the second toe, then repeat the bicycling motion until you have pressed each toe in the same manner. If another parent is available to help, have them place their hand gently on the lower belly while you do these movements on the toes.

Yawning. This is a great sign and, just like rubbing of the eyes, it means that you have turned on the relaxation response in your child's body. (See also **Eye rubbing**.)

Relax-Relate Cues vs Stress Cues

Table 9.1 Reading body cues – quick reference chart

Relax-Relate Responses	Stress Responses
Hums	Pushes hands away
Sighs	Runs away
Yawns	Avoids touch in any area
Makes eye contact	Avoids eye contact
Rubs eyes	Head up
Hand on your hand	Knees up
Far-off relaxed stare	Heels up
Lays down	Ticklish
Relaxes head down	Winces in pain

Always Another Chance

It will take a while until your response to all of these body cues becomes second nature. Stay calm when you get an anxious response during the movements and keep this book nearby so you can easily look things up. If you have another parent doing QST with you, you can talk things over as you go, and one of you can look things up while the other continues calmly working with your child. While it is important that you diligently try to learn as much as you can from this handbook and that you refresh your knowledge by reading it repeatedly in the early weeks, you can't expect to know everything at first. If you missed a response and you didn't get to deal with something in the optimal way on a certain day, remember that *your child will always give you another chance!* After all, if the block is still there, you can clear it another day. In the meantime, it is more important to be patient with yourself, relax and enjoy the time with your child.

Chapter 10

How to Work Through the Difficult Spots

When beginning QST, because it is a new form of stimulation, it's not unusual for children to find ingenious and often exasperating ways to resist and avoid the routine, ways that can disrupt your own rhythm and even derail your efforts. This chapter gives you a set of tools to successfully address and resolve these disruptions, including any doubts that may arise for you as you do the movements. By using some of the same skills you have already learned, we provide a 'how-to' of what to do if you are met with common kinds of resistance and avoidance and help you to see these derailing behaviors through the lens of sensory overload and restoration. As you will see in the next chapter (Chapter 11), these are the very same QST skills that you will soon learn to use *outside* of QST, anytime and anywhere you want to help your child regulate difficult behaviors during the day. But first, let's begin with how to address disruptions and impediments *while doing* the routine itself.

Your Child's Resistance to QST

If you feel that your child's resistance is deeper, stronger or more problematic than simply voicing objections to mild discomfort and he doesn't respond to variations you try with your touch, there are several things that might be going on. The following are common resistances you may encounter, the meanings behind them and what you can do to help. This is not always easy in the moment, but over time, you will get better and better at it.

Fight or flight. If at any point in the routine you believe you've activated your child's survival mode – he pushes you away, refuses your touch, or even possibly screams and/or fiercely resists – it can mean that the new and confusing sensations have probably triggered a fight-or-flight reaction. When he is in this sensory overload, his thinking brain shuts down, and he is literally not hearing your words. He is a captive of his survival brain. In those moments, it is very important *not to restrain him* or get into a struggle, as this will only intensify the experience of threat. Remember, the fight-flight response is an automatic and spontaneous reaction to the sensory overload he is experiencing. It is not bad behavior, and it is *not* willful. He needs your calm, confident,

DOI: 10.4324/9781003360421-13

co-regulating presence. Establishing a sense of safety begins with your own awareness. The following suggestions will help you find what works best in the moment:

- Stop the QST movement that triggered his reaction and take a moment to find your own breath. You don't have to rush; your child's brain will register your shift and *even that shift can start the process of down-regulating* both your nervous system and his.
- Then find a way to confidently and safely *contain – not restrain –* him. This can take many forms. Often, quieting your hands right where they are in the movement and letting them rest warmly and quietly on your child's body will be enough. Or it can be a reassuring touch or hug. We find that once parents find their own calm, they know just what will work best in the moment. Your soothing tone of voice and confident and regulating touch will lend him your calm.
- If his fight-flight response is so heightened that any form of touch makes it worse, move your hands away. But know that in this moment, he needs your reassuring presence more than ever. Sometimes it is through your silent but resolved presence that he knows you are there and are giving him the time and space he needs – that you both need – to quiet your nervous systems.

Once you have helped him out of the spontaneous fight-flight response, you can resume the movements right where you left off. In the early weeks of QST, this may require short breaks. Your calm presence and your attuned and patient touch will help him to tolerate the routine for longer and longer periods without triggering this spontaneous sensory overwhelm. Take it slowly and patiently. He will respond.

Avoidance without agitation. If your child runs away from the treatment but isn't necessarily agitated, it will help to have both parents involved. One can hold and *contain* the child on his or her lap while the other does the QST movements. But if you are doing this alone, it's perfectly okay if you have to follow the child to where he is and continue the movements from whatever position he comes to rest in, whether sitting, standing or laying down. Do the movement the best you can. If he continues to flee after trying this a couple of times, you can stop and wait for a time when he is more receptive and begin the treatment again with the same movement where you left off, doing a few movements at a time. Over time, you'll be able to get more and more of the movements done, until he is finally able to tolerate all 12 steps at once.

Refusal to lie down. When a child refuses to lie on his belly for Movements 5 and 6, it can mean there is a block in the belly. These are not literal blocks in the belly per se; they are blocks to the channels that send energy, as understood by Chinese medicine, to the digestive system so it can work properly. You might need to do more of Movements 3 and 4 to clear the belly before he turns over and you start the movements down the back. Another reason your child may refuse to lie down, either on his back or tummy, is that there is a block in the head and energy is not able to flow downward toward the hands and feet. In this situation, you can do the movement with your child standing up or sitting. Once he starts to relax, you will be able to guide him to lie down.

Fearful agitation. Sometimes, children simply get upset and fearful when they are faced with new sensations and feelings. There are two additional specific techniques that can help. Both of these involve the help of a second partner. If that is not possible for you, we've made note how to accomplish the same goal by yourself.

- Some children feel extra support when one partner holds them gently while the other does the movement. Try sitting your child in one parent's lap (child facing out, his back nestled against parent's chest) with parent's arms wrapped around him. Nestling against somebody's chest can be very comforting. This gives your child a sense of contained safety without being restrained, while your reassuring words and your actions convey that he can trust you to help. Make sure to complete the movements right over the top of the holding parent's hands so as not to disrupt the energy flow of the movement.
- A second approach that sometimes helps calm a frightened child is to have your partner press gently on the top of your child's head, using a relaxed palm and a rhythmic pressing movement as you are giving the QST. Here again, you should complete the movements over the top of the hands of the parent who is holding the child so as not to disrupt the energy flow.
- If alone, nestle your child in your lap or on your chest in the same manner until he quiets. From this position, you can use the same gentle, rhythmic pressing movement on the top of his head as above. You may have to begin with just your hand resting warmly and confidently on top of your child's head, then slowly introduce the gentle rhythmic pressing movement.

Resistance in toddlers. A toddler's will is just emerging and is extremely strong. Add to that an immature sensory nervous system that puts extra stress on a toddler's energy, and it isn't uncommon for him to complain loudly about your first attempts to give QST. We have found that most toddlers will put up quite a fuss for the first week or so, but the fuss is mostly vocal (not fighting with arms and legs). As long as his body is relatively quiet – and relative is an important word when talking about toddlers being still – this is his will expressing itself, not a fight-or-flight response. In this situation, one parent holds him in a way to provide safe containment *without forcefully restraining*, while the other parent does the steps of the routine. If you don't have access to another caregiver, you can do this equally well by slowing down and taking cuddle breaks to bring him back to calm.

Questions to Ask Yourself When Stuck

As you address some of these resistances, it is common to have some normal doubts and questions. After all, you are doing something new and possibly uncomfortable for both of you. This is the time when parents can get frustrated and overwhelmed themselves or even feel tempted to give up. If you feel stuck in this way, don't give up! Give yourself a break and ask yourself the following three questions. The answers and awareness they provide often help you get back on track.

1. Am I Doing QST Correctly?

The best way to answer this question is to review the *QST Sensory Movement Chart* once again [Appendix A]. If you feel unsure, see if you can try the movements on your spouse or a friend. Ask them if the routine felt relaxing and enjoyable. Make note of any problem areas. If you don't have someone to work with, watch the online videos again to make sure what you are doing matches the steps in the video. Here are some questions to ask yourself about your technique:

- Are your hands starting and ending in the right places?
- Are you carefully following the channels as shown by the lines on the *QST Sensory Movement Chart?*
- Is your child in a comfortable place and are you able to perform the routine easily and comfortably in the space you are using?
- Are you patting too hard or with a flat hand? Try patting faster and lighter or, if that doesn't help, go with slower, deeper pressure. In the online videos, pay close attention to the weight of the hand being used in the motions. A general rule is to pat with the weight you would use when burping an infant, firm but comforting.

2. Am I Staying Calm and Relaxed?

QST works best when you begin at a calm and relaxed place yourself. Each parent knows what works best for them, whether it's taking a few quiet breaths to slow down the busyness of the day or rubbing your hands together to feel the warmth of the loving energy that you will send to your child. If you are ill, exhausted, upset, tense or angry, this will communicate itself to your child and a good treatment routine will not be possible.

3. Am I Doing the QST Movements Too Quickly?

You can do everything else right, but if you rush too quickly, it can over-stimulate rather than calm your child's nervous system. Parents are often surprised to find that all they need to do is slow down (see "Slow is Key" in Chapter 5, page 42) and the most important question to ask at that point is: Am I rushing, either in my movements or in my responses? You can even stop for a moment, resting the warmth of your palms in place on your child right where you are doing the movement, take a deep relaxing breath in and a slow exhale for yourself, then resume with the slower, rhythmic pace once your child has settled. It's better to do the movements in a relaxed way and only complete some of them than try to rush to get them all in. If your child needs a break, you can always complete the rest at another time.

Do I need to switch from patting to pressing? Switching from patting to pressing is another basic skill that many parents tend to forget when their child resists or fusses. For example, we may remember to slow down but forget to switch to pressing. Then we wonder what's wrong. It helps to remember this simple rule: a hyper-sensitive child may not tolerate the patting movement in the beginning and may require a different touch technique. Instead of patting, try gently pressing through all of the movements until your child can begin to tolerate patting. You do ultimately want his body to tolerate gentle patting, but you may have to work your way up to that. So, if patting is a problem, switching to slower pressing can be a highly effective way to reduce your child's sensitivity.

Is my child completely unable to accept QST? For some children who are not in the fight-or-flight state, you can go slowly and pat as quickly and lightly as you can, but he still may not tolerate the movements. In these instances, the problem is often a blocking of energy in the head area. You may need to do more de-blocking movements for the head/neck (see Chapter 8, page 76 – Extra Neck Clearing) because it will be difficult to complete all 12 QST movements until his head feels more comfortable. Try the following approaches, one at a time:

- Start Movement 5 at the base of the head, trying to clear some of the blocks there and below before going back to the top of the head.
- Do the first part of Movement 5 in the air above the head (that is, do it a few inches above but do not touch the head) and then continue down the body in the same way for the first week.
- For the first week, limit the QST to the first three movements and do them several times a day, quickly and lightly.
- Try doing QST while he is watching a video in the beginning.
- Break the QST into parts and only do a few movements each day.
- Try doing some of the movements on your child's body while he is asleep.

In Summary

Whatever your questions or hesitations, follow these simple guidelines:

- Be gentle.
- Don't continue QST through fight or flight.
- Make sure you both are comfortable.
- Do the routine once daily.
- Do the movements from the top down.

If you do these things, you have little to fear. You will not make your child worse. Even incremental improvement is well worth the effort.

Additional Resources for Help

Sometimes you try everything and still feel at an impasse. Turn to Appendix D – Getting Personalized QST Help (page 211), where you'll find information on how to find a Certified QST Trainer in your local area or arrange a Zoom/Skype or other online consultation.

QST for Everyday 'Challenging' Behaviors

In this chapter, we take the insights and touch techniques that you have learned in QST and show you how to use those skills anytime or anywhere that 'difficult behaviors' arise in daily life. Whether it's a meltdown at the supermarket, aggression or a tantrum while playing with friends, freezing in place when asked to stop a game and come to the dinner table – whatever the stress behavior or sensory overload, you now have a new set of skills to take with you and use during the course of your daily activities. All you need to do is what you've already been doing in the routine: look under the behavior, identify the sensory overload and use your touch to foster regulation and transitions back to the calm receptive state. The guidelines you'll find in the pages ahead show you how to apply those skills in specific, everyday behavioral situations.

Be a Stress Detective

At times when your child exhibits difficult behaviors, it can help to think of yourself as what Dr. Stuart Shanker (2016) has termed a "stress detective". Your job is to find the clues to the causes of the stress and eliminate or reduce them. This opens the door to more effective strategies. A good detective needs to know what to pay attention to and what kinds of hidden details might point to the real causes. So, let's get out our magnifying glass and take a look at some of the hidden causes of your child's challenging behaviors.

Common Causes of Challenging Behaviors

There are four broad causes that commonly stress a child's sensory system and lead to challenging behaviors. They are:

1. Physical problems
2. Communication difficulties
3. Lack of specific skills or maturation
4. Problems with behavioral self-regulation

Each of these sources of stress is different and has its own distinct set of solutions. That makes it very important to have a pretty good idea of what you are trying to fix before you attempt to fix

DOI: 10.4324/9781003360421-14

it. Let's take a look at each stressor, how to identify it and what you can do to reduce the load on your child's sensory system.

Physical problems. The first place to look for any child in distress, but especially for one with a sensory problem, is the possibility of a physical stressor. Your child may be tired, hungry, too hot, too cold, or bothered by lights, noise or even discomfort from her clothes or diaper. In fact, a child can be uncomfortable or in distress for any number of reasons that a parent may not be aware of. But as any good detective will tell you, the first place to look should be right under your own nose! And the answer can be just as simple as eliminating the cause by feeding your child if hungry or removing the discomfort.

With physical problems, notice if the behaviors happen at the same time of day. When that happens, think about changing the daily routine to eliminate the problem. Still, some environments like certain play areas, malls or stores have too many people, too much noise, light that is too bright or are simply too busy and chaotic for your child to function without having to shut down. In these cases, it is best to try to keep your child away from those areas when you can. Finally, don't forget that sensory overload can magnify the response to a physical problem. Under stress, your child's body is awash with the release of stress hormones and the bodily reactions they cause. That burns a lot of energy and means that even with the best of responses from you, it can take some time for your child to return to being calm and receptive once triggered.

Communication difficulties. A second basic clue to the cause of stress behavior has to do with communication: your child may simply not understand or comprehend what you are telling her. She may have congestion or fluid in her ears. Some children may have language delay which might mean that they can hear but not fully understand what you are asking them to do. And don't forget what we talked about in Chapter 1, stress can literally cause changes in the inner ear restricting the range of what your child can hear when she is in survival mode. If you have a question about whether your child can hear or understand you, pay close attention to her face and behavior to see whether she understands. If it looks like she doesn't, then slow down and simplify the instruction. Complicated sentences tend to overwhelm a sensory child, and repeating yourself is futile if she doesn't understand you in the first place. And talking louder will only amp up the stress for both of you. Instead, use fewer and simpler words, even three-word sentences or non-verbal commands. Break down the request into smaller, easy-to-comprehend parts and be sure to offer support through each of the steps until you are sure she understands.

Lacking required skills or maturation. Most inabilities due to delayed maturity are easy to spot; you wouldn't ask a toddler to ride a bike because she is not developmentally ready for that complex task. But there are many other more subtle skills that are harder to see. For example, certain social and emotional skills are required to understand how to play well with others. Language processing skills are required for a child to understand what she is being told, while other skills help to express wants, frustrations or displeasure. Also, as we'll see later, sensory kids often lack the processing, sequence and delay of impulse skills necessary to manage smooth transitions from one activity to another. Some of these skills may not have yet kicked in developmentally. That will require some patience on your part and maybe a work-around that helps your child process or do what's needed in a different or simpler way. Remember, a good detective will always make sure to not ask a child to do what she really can't yet do.

Problems with behavioral self-regulation. Because stress behavior can go on and on and appear to be willful, it's easy to think that your child is just being stubborn. But that overlooks one of the most important clues to her actions, her inability to regulate her own feelings and emotions. As we discussed in Chapter 2, a child must achieve the four self-regulatory milestones, usually in the first two years – regulated sleep, digestion, attention and the ability to self-soothe – before she can start to learn to regulate her behavior by the third and fourth years. If your child has missed one or more of these four milestones, she misses the basic building blocks to learn to regulate her behavior as she gets older, and she'll need your help to go back to recapture those basic abilities.

Think about those milestones whenever you see a challenging behavior and ask yourself what self-regulatory stepping stone may need your help. For example, some challenging behaviors that at first look like a problem with communication skills may turn out to be a problem with the attention milestone. Irritable behavior may be caused by physical discomfort, or it may relate to a missed milestone of regulated sleep, digestion or self-soothing. Behaviors that may look like impaired social or emotional skills may actually be your child's unregulated reaction to the strong feelings or emotions of the people around her. Finding the right cause is not always easy. You will need to look in the most obvious of places (physical causes) and in the subtlest (self-regulatory milestones). Then, you will see challenging behaviors through new eyes and with new choices of action.

QST Skills for Challenging Behaviors

Now that you're thinking like a stress detective, you can put the puzzle pieces together, look *under* the behavior to see its deeper causes and target your intentions and actions to reduce it. In the quick-reference section below (Table 11.1), we've listed several of the most common stress behaviors, clues to some of their probable causes and some helpful actions to reduce the stress. This list includes typical behaviors for most 3- and 4-year-olds and reflects normal developmental responses for children of this age. When looking for stressors, there can sometimes be more than one. Not every reaction is a result of a child's problem. Sometimes, especially for younger children, you may be seeing normal reactions for that developmental age. But when you see these same behaviors in older children, say six years or older, they often reflect an immature sensory system. Don't despair! Most children can catch up developmentally if given the right help. When you can identify the missed self-regulatory milestones and help restore them through QST, you will re-set your child on the path to more mature growth.

Once you can more easily spot the common underlying causes and solutions to typical challenging behaviors, there will still always be those times that leave you stuck or baffled. We have had a lot of experience with parents of sensory kids and have put together a useful set of tools for just these occasions. We start with some specific and often very difficult behaviors such as kicking and biting. Parents are sometimes surprised to learn that many of these very difficult behaviors are responsive to the same techniques that they have already used in the daily routine. We have adapted some of those skills for you to use in those daily dysregulated and challenging moments. They are *not* intended to control behavior. They are designed to help you reduce your child's stress by creating a sense of safety and connection to you so that, in time, she can come to regulate her own behavior.

Table 11.1 Challenging behaviors – quick reference guide:
Difficult behaviors that are triggered by stress.

Aggression is commonly a consequence of sensory stress overload, a lack of communication skills and/ or hyperactivity from sugar overload or food triggers.
  Solutions
  - Identify and minimize environments that trigger sensory overload (e.g., shopping right after school or work, play areas in fast food restaurants.)
  - Eliminate food triggers (e.g., sugars, red dye in food.)
  - See: *Aggressive Behaviors – Hitting-Kicking-Biting* later in this chapter for skills to address these issues specifically.

Not listening is often caused by hearing problems, communication difficulties such as not understanding the request or a skill that is too difficult for her to do on her own.
  Solutions
  - Put special focus on Movement 8 (ear to hand) and extra neck and ear clearing to help the ears drain, supporting language development and maturation of the attention milestone.
  - Break down the request into small steps the child can understand.

Doing the opposite of what was asked may simply be caused by not understanding the instruction. Be sure to make room for oppositional behavior, which is a normal step toward autonomy.
  Solutions
  - Were directions clear, or were they given too quickly or too many words?
  - See *Refusing to cooperate* in this list below. Also see *Teaching Simple Directions* later in this chapter.

Planting (sitting down) and refusing to move can be a sign that your child is moving into overwhelm or freeze mode. It is important to consider causes such as an environment that is too overwhelming, a task that is too difficult, hard-to-understand directions or physical exhaustion.
  Solutions
  - Simplify requests so they are doable. Remove from over-stimulating environments.
  - Perform daily QST to improve language, attention and self-soothing.

Refusing to cooperate can be caused by a delay of early attention and self-soothing milestones. Or it may indicate that your child has entered freeze mode.
  Solutions
  - Focus on Movement 2 (relax chest) to help the attention and self-soothing milestones.
  - To manage freeze mode, see *Planting and refusing to move* earlier.

Running away from you can result from basic problems in communication skills. Your child hasn't learned "Stop!" and "Come to Mommy". This skill must be learned at home first.
  Solutions
  - Focus on simple safety commands.
  - Teach the skills in the quiet, protected environment of the home.

Temper tantrums are most often related to a delay in the self-soothing milestone.
  Solutions
  - Focus on Movement 2 (relax chest) to reduce the frequency and duration of tantrums while developing the self-soothing milestone.

Difficulties with transitions are frequently caused by a delay in the self-soothing milestone.
  Solutions
  - Focus on Movement 2 (relax chest) to develop self-soothing skills.
  - See **Help with transitions**, later in chapter.

Wandering off is often brought on by lack of awareness of a danger or lack of body awareness.
  Solutions
  - Develop a safety plan (e.g., locks on doors, etc.)
  - Perform daily QST to develop body awareness

Aggressive Behaviors: Hitting-Kicking-Biting

Sensory kids can easily be tipped into survival mode, which can result in all sorts of aggressive behaviors including pinching, hitting, kicking, biting and even spitting. These behaviors are usually triggered very quickly, sometimes with only a one- or two-second warning. While they may at first look to you like basic aggression, they are actually the knee-jerk response (fight mode) of an immature nervous system that hasn't yet had the opportunity to learn to deal appropriately with pain, threat or frustration. They reflect self-defense more than real aggression and are commonly triggered by one of three things:

1. Touch feels painful
2. Her personal space has been invaded too quickly
3. Her wishes and needs are frustrated or something that belongs to her has been taken away

With each of the following techniques, your calm, intentional touch will stop the behavior and dial down the fight-flight part of your child's brain. But you must act *quickly*. This technique won't work if you try it 5 or 10 minutes after the aggressive behavior has started, and it certainly won't work if you get upset yourself. Your child's brain is in survival mode and tuned not to your spoken words but to the *tone* of your voice, the *expression* on your face and the *tension* in your body posture. So, your first step is to calm yourself with a deep breath in and slow exhale out. And quietly focus your intention on the following course of action.

Hitting or pinching: Immediately reach out and firmly but gently squeeze the hand that pinched or hit and say in a *calm*, firm voice, "No hitting [pinching]. Gentle hands." This will probably surprise your child, but if your voice stays calm and your expression is soft but resolute, your firm pressure will re-focus her awareness on to her body and help to switch her brain over into receptive mode. At that point, she will be able to hear you. Continue this firm pressure until you feel her hands relax.

Kicking: The moment your child kicks, take both feet in your hands, squeeze them firmly but gently and say in a clear, *calm* voice, "No kicking. Gentle feet." If she is lying down, put gentle pressure above both knees and say the same thing. Continue until she relaxes her legs.

Biting or spitting: Firmly press down on both shoulders at the same time, then firmly but gently squeeze down the arms to the hands while saying in a clear and calm voice, "No biting [spitting]. Gentle." Repeat this several times, holding her hands firmly in yours.

These behaviors will usually stop immediately. If your child is verbal, you can also talk with her about what just happened and encourage her to use her words instead. For the less verbal child, you may say, "When we are frustrated, we use our words." But if she is primarily non-verbal, it is often enough to just stop the behavior. While the frequency of these behaviors tends to drop quickly, you may need to repeat these actions several times. Your firm tone of voice and calm expression are very important for success because your child's nervous system is exquisitely tuned to even the slightest signal of threat. While doing this won't always be easy in the heat of the moment, you will find that it comes more naturally as you help your child become more receptive.

Help with Transitions

It isn't easy for sensory kids to make smooth transitions. Once their nervous system is accustomed to one activity, it can be very disturbing to change. In fact, you probably already have run into this problem the moment you asked your child to stop playing and get ready for QST. She may well have resisted, even though she enjoys the treatment. Why? Because change isn't easy for her, and it is here that she needs your extra support. To make that smooth transition, she must first be able to listen and pay attention to what is expected. To do that, she needs to remain calm and open so she can give up one thing and start the next.

When your child has problems with transitions, you understandably can feel frustrated and helpless. You may try to bribe or bargain with her to cooperate. "If you come with me to pick up your sister, I'll give you a candy bar." But bribing and bargaining are only temporary solutions, and there are educational, social and emotional transitions ahead that she will need to smoothly navigate. Helping her today will pave the way for those larger transitions of the future.

We've adapted a rather simple and effective technique to help her focus her attention and keep her calm. As we've said, this technique works best once you can trigger the self-soothing relaxation response in Movement 2 on the chest. In other words, she has to have first learned to relax with pressure on her chest. Let's start with an example. Say your child is watching TV and you want her to come to the dinner table. *Here's what you do*:

1. **Make a connection with touch.** Sit next to her without saying anything. Place one hand on the front of her chest and the other hand on her back directly behind her chest. Make a firm and gentle connection. This will get her attention and feel soothing at the same time.
2. **Give the instruction.** When you have her attention, tell her what will happen next: "It's time to eat dinner".
3. **Repeat and offer help.** If she doesn't respond or start to move on her own, repeat, "It's time to come and eat dinner", and ask if she needs help.
4. **Give physical guidance.** If she still doesn't respond, keep a steady hold (back and front) on her chest and gently but firmly guide her upright saying, "Let's go and eat dinner." Walk next to her keeping the physical contact with her chest between your hands until she sees the dinner table and her chair. At that point, she should be able to complete the transition and sit down in her chair for dinner [also see online video: *QST-Making Transitions Easier* link in Appendix H].

While this may sound simple, it can be very effective, and you'll be surprised how much better it works than just telling her to come to dinner. Actually, most children do like to eat dinner. But change for sensory kids can be very difficult and threatening. When you place pressure on her chest and her back, you re-trigger that self-soothing response that you have been developing and strengthening over these many weeks. It is that extra support that helps her to feel calm while she switches from doing one thing and transitions to the next. With time, you'll be able to achieve the same result with only a firm and gentle hand on the middle of her back.

Dealing With Sitting and Planting

Sitting and planting behavior occurs when your child slows down, plants herself in a seated position and does not move. Children who do this are often unfairly labeled stubborn, inflexible or oppositional. But stubbornness would involve a decision to oppose you, and the sensory child isn't able to decide anything at all. Her thinking brain has shut down and she can't listen, think or move. This is overload or freeze mode, and the physical signs are slowed movement, sitting down and planting, loss of facial expression, staring and loss of eye contact. When you see this happening, you've lost contact with your child. How you handle it will make all the difference. Here's how to help:

- First, if you feel yourself getting upset, take a moment to calm down and remember that her brain needs your physical reassurance to know she is safe.
- Then pick her up and hold her lovingly in your lap.
- Talk softly to her, reassuring her that she is OK. Your tone and inflection are what count, words are less important. Do not expect an answer.
- Physical contact with you works best for most children, most of the time. Your child's nervous system needs to down-regulate out of freeze mode, and her body needs a chance to wash the stress hormones out of her system. This can take time. However, if physical contact at this moment triggers a stress response, just sit quietly without touching. Your silent calm presence will be reassuring until she is ready for contact or engagement.
- Once you feel her body start to relax, you can cover her with a blanket, give her a favorite toy and let her relax until she is ready to rejoin the previous activities. Remember stress uses a lot of energy and she may need some downtime to recover.

It is important to respond to sitting and planting in a helpful way rather than seeing it only as stubborn or oppositional behavior. That's because if your child repeatedly gets stuck in overwhelm mode, she will learn to avoid new learning situations. We want her to be confident when she goes to school and comfortable when she learns new things. This technique will help her to get started down that road.

QST Skills for Every Day

QST skills are adaptable for all occasions. As you become more comfortable with the routine, you will find that these skills become part of your everyday activities and that you can use them to help your child whether she is sitting, standing or walking – anytime, anywhere you see that your child's nervous system is winding up and sensory overload has begun to intensify her behaviors. Here are some more general techniques that you can add to your toolbox whenever your child needs help to self-regulate.

Teaching Simple Directions

There are many reasons, not least of which is safety, why every child needs to learn to follow simple instructions at home. For sensory children, learning this skill can take a little more work, but in time it will become central to success in school. That's why we suggest these simple steps:

- **Make a touch connection** with your child (stroke her back, take her hands in yours, sit her in your lap). That will get her attention so she can be more receptive to verbal instructions.
- **Make eye contact** to be sure you have her attention and that she understands.
- **Connect** with her verbally by saying her name.
- **Explain** what needs to happen using as few words as possible, e.g., "Shoes on".
- **Offer her a choice** such as, "Do you need help with . . . ?"
- **Remain engaged** with her until she succeeds in following the instruction.
- **Avoid over-using the word 'no'** If everything is a 'no', why obey? Save "No!" for safety issues such as not going near a hot stove or electrical outlet. When you do say "No!", your tone and inflection are more important than your words. Your child needs to know you are serious but *not* angry or afraid. To accomplish that, make sure your breath is slower and deeper. Your voice must be calm and slow but resolute.

'Mini QST'

This simple technique came out of our work with young children with autism. It is adapted from some of the same movements you use in the QST sensory routine. These short techniques are designed to deal with a stress response right where it is happening and enable your child to make these otherwise simple transitions. *Here's what to do:*

1. When you see your child's shoulders lifting as a result of stress, just pat the top of them like you would do in Movement 7 (down the sides). Keep patting until the shoulders loosen.
2. Then, squeeze down her arms like you would in Movement 1 until both the shoulders and arms relax.
3. You can finish this short technique with some long calming strokes down her back.

These three brief movements will only take a few minutes and can be a very effective tool under all kinds of circumstances. This technique will work best once you have some success with Movement 2 on the chest and are able to trigger her self-soothing response (rubbing eyes, yawning). You'll also find that as you learn your child's own signals of body tension, you'll be able to react more quickly to stop the flood of stress hormones before fight-flight-or-freeze locks into place and to quiet those tensions before they accumulate. In time, she will learn to turn to you for reassurance when she begins to feel stressed.

Challenging Your Child: Good Stress and Bad Stress

On a final note, don't forget that as you are *being challenged* by your child, it is also your job to supportively *challenge her* in just the right ways. To grow, your child needs to develop a base of experience and a history of success with new tasks that will always be just slightly above her level of ability. While we've talked throughout this book about how stress disrupts behavior, remember that some stress is necessary and positive. It feels stressful when we are expected to do something we've never done before. Healthy stress is essential for growth and good development. That means that a good stress detective learns and responds differently to good versus bad stress.

When you spot good stress situations, gently challenge your child toward new growth by breaking the stressful task into small manageable steps while you provide support so she can experience success and develop confidence. When you present her with the right kind of support and graduated challenge, you help her to avoid overwhelm mode. Then she can start to build the self-regulation capacities that allow her to master new learning situations. *Most importantly, she'll learn that bad stress can be managed while good stress can be welcomed.* In time, she will no longer need to avoid new tasks or situations, school will be a fun place to learn and she'll have the self-regulation skills that she will use for the rest of her life.

Bibliography

Chapter 11

Shanker, S., & Barker, T. (2016). Eat, play, sleep: The biological domain. In *Self-Reg: How to Help Your Child (and You) Break the Stress Cycle and Successfully Engage with Life*, Penguin Random House, New York, 97.

Chapter 12

Optimizing Diet, Nutrition and Daily Routines

This final chapter addresses the other essential building blocks to healthy development that are often overlooked in busy lives today – diet, sleep and rhythmic daily routines. We'll look at how you – with a few simple improvements in what food you make, how you provide for sleep and rest, which toxins and allergens you avoid and how you organize your day – can build upon the success you have with QST. These changes will target those easily forgotten parts of the day that may act as hidden triggers that contribute to your child's symptoms.

Diet and Nutrition

Current research clearly shows that the health of the gut and digestive system is essential for healthy development. We now know that the delicate balance of bacteria in the intestines, known as the gut microbiome, has a direct influence not only on gastrointestinal and digestive heath but also on brain function, the strength of the immune and endocrine systems and cognitive, emotional and behavioral health. Neurotransmitters from the gut microbiome have been shown to directly impact mood, anxiety-like symptoms and hyperactivity. This is especially true for your sensory child, whose immature nervous system is often linked to a weaker and less mature digestive system than would be typical for her age. Gut imbalances can also lead to many gastrointestinal problems including poor appetite, constipation, diarrhea and a determination to eat only a very narrow range of foods.

Perspectives from Chinese Medicine

There is a wealth of valuable information about nutritional and dietary advice for parents today, and while some of it can be frustratingly complicated and contradictory, there is a great deal there to help you find the diet that is right for your child. It is not our purpose to recommend any specific diet because every sensory child is unique in their reaction to food. Instead, we offer something different, a view from Chinese medicine about how to feed a young child with developmental challenges and a set of general principles that we think will be beneficial no matter what diet you choose.

A child with a strong digestive system will have a good appetite and normal bowels. But sensory kids often have poor appetites and bowel problems which are markers of a weak digestive system. You can think of your digestive system, from the perspective of Chinese medicine, as a kind of slow cooker that processes your food and extracts the nutrition from it. This perspective gives us some

DOI: 10.4324/9781003360421-15

good guidelines on how to prepare our food, what to avoid and how to look for signs that a child's slow cooker is either doing its job or needs our assistance. The focus here is on the quality of food, how to prepare it and what to avoid. When all that is working well, you should expect to see not only improvements in your child's sensory symptoms but, more importantly, signs that those most basic roots of self-regulation – digestion, sleep and elimination – have gotten back on a healthy track. Here are some simple, common-sense principals to follow that have worked for centuries.

Food Should be Warm and Cooked

How you prepare food so your child can best digest it is just as important as what food you choose. For example, you wouldn't feed an infant iced smoothies with raw vegetables – that would surely lead to tummy aches and diarrhea, and the nutrients would pass right out the other end. You would cook the food, puree it and warm it up. But what is easy to see with an infant is not always as clear cut for an older child. Think again about our slow cooker. Cold foods will take longer to heat up in order to be digested, and others, like raw vegetables, may simply just take longer to digest. That means that both the temperature and the type of food you offer are important to keep in mind.

Digestion takes a lot of energy, and if your child isn't digesting well, cold food will only make things worse. Your child will have to use what little digestive energy she has to warm up the food and then 'cook' or digest it. A lot of times we unknowingly make it harder for our children to digest their food by feeding them iced or cold food. First of all, ice slows everything down. The stomach is a muscle, and if you ice a muscle, it gets stiff and stops working. None of the digestive enzymes work at cold or freezing temperatures, they only work at body temperature, so the body has to take what little energy it has for digestion and use it to melt the ice. Then it has to take more energy to warm up the food so the enzymes can work.

Raw vegetables can also slow digestion because it takes the stomach a long time and a lot of energy to digest them. Think how long it takes to cook vegetables on the stove. In fact, when it comes to feeding your child raw vegetables, we feel that the food pyramid diet plan that is usually recommended for children is almost never right for a child with digestive problems. The plan recommends too much cold and raw food for your child's weaker digestive system and energy needs. What's needed is nutritious food that is easy to digest and will allow her to get the nutrition she needs without her system having to work too hard. So, here are *three simple rules about food preparation* that make digestion easier for children with sensory and/or developmental problems.

1. Stay away from ice.
2. Warm up the food.
3. Cook all vegetables.

These rules have been around for a long time, and while they may sound new to parents in the United States, they are well known to Asian and European parents. Follow them, along with your QST daily routine, and within a few months, we think you will find your child eating more and even beginning to sample foods that she had never tried before.

What Foods Should I Feed My Child?

You want your child to enjoy meals, eat regularly, be satisfied and not overeat. You want the meals to be nutritious and to provide lots of readily available energy. Although fast food and sugar provide quick energy, they have lots of preservatives, artificial flavoring and stronger flavors than natural food. The strong flavors interfere with your child's appetite and can trigger cravings for sugar. They can also lead to weight problems. For all these reasons, it's best to stay away from processed food, sweets, candy and fast food. Most importantly, children need to develop the feeling for what foods are good and how much is enough. This will happen naturally if you avoid processed and sugary foods and go with simple, warm, homemade foods. *Here are some guidelines for what to prepare:*

- Simple, warm, homemade meals three times a day, as much as possible
- Cooked vegetables
- Cooked grains/starches such as oatmeal, rice and noodles
- Proteins such as meat or fish (or healthy substitute for meatless diets)
- Whole, fresh fruit and berries for snacks
- Avoid processed food, fast food, artificial colors, artificial flavors and foods high in sugar
- Water (room temperature) to drink with each meal instead of the variety of sweetened juices and milk products that are available

Should I Limit Milk Products?

You'll notice we didn't include milk products in the guidelines above. Milk products include milk, ice cream, yogurt and cheese. For many children with sensory and developmental problems, milk products stimulate mucus production and lead to sinus congestion and problems with the ears. If your child has a lot of mucus congestion, she is likely to benefit from cutting out milk products completely for three months as you first switch her diet to all warm and cooked food. Once the mucus is gone, you can try introducing a little milk or yogurt one to three times a week and observe closely. If the mucus doesn't come back, you can add a little more. If it does, you will have to cut out milk products again. Mucus congestion can plug your child's ears, so continuing foods that produce mucus can create a risk to hearing and speech. For information about foods you can substitute for dairy in young children, local parent support groups and internet groups can be very helpful.

Other Food Intolerances and Allergies?

The best way to deal with food intolerances and allergies is, of course, to take steps to avoid them. If your child has been receiving the wrong diet and has had reflux, diarrhea or constipation for some time, the digestive tract can get irritated and develop problems digesting foods such as wheat, eggs, nuts, dairy or citrus. Once the diet is switched to warm and cooked foods, the overall situation will improve. Sometimes, a problem with a particular food will stand out. In that case, as with dairy, remove the food for three months and then re-introduce it slowly in small, infrequent amounts. In some cases, parents have also removed all genetically modified food from their children's diets with good results.

Signs That My Child Is Having Difficulty Digesting Food

If your child enjoys meals, eats a variety of foods and doesn't overeat or show any digestive problems, then the food she is eating is probably digesting well. However, there are immediate and long-term signs that a child isn't digesting well. Constipation, diarrhea, undigested food in bowel movements, reflux, tummy aches, eczema, sweet cravings and/or mucus congestion – and yes, behavioral problems – can all signal problems with diet and digestion. For example, we have seen children develop reflux within days of being given iced fruit smoothies in the morning and have seen that reflux stop just as quickly when the smoothies were stopped. With longer-term use of cold food, we have seen the whole digestive system slow down and children become constipated. If this is the reason for the constipation, it can be reversed quickly. As it turns out, the solutions to many of these digestive problems can be quite simple, including avoiding cold and raw food, eliminating ice drinks, reducing sugar and alertness to the impact of milk products. Your child will have more energy for growth and development. If problems persist, your pediatrician can test to see if there is a medical and/or structural problem that is affecting digestion.

A Note About Toxicity

In our world today, we are all vulnerable to accumulating some toxins. But since most are invisible to us, it can be hard to understand how they can build up in our bodies and how that process can block the free flow of energy and nutrients to our organ systems. We only become aware of these effects indirectly through physical symptoms, illness and mood or behavioral problems. We can reduce this toxic load for our children by watching what we feed them, what products we use and what substances we avoid. To better understand how toxins build up, visualize a river. Our bodies, like a river, can absorb some amount of toxins before becoming polluted. They have a 'carrying capacity', or an ability to carry away waste and still remain healthy. But if that carrying capacity is exceeded, the river becomes toxic, the fish that live in it become ill and the land around it suffers. The river slows down and trash collects in the bends and twists, plugging the entry and exit points. The same is true for the channels in your child's body that carry qi-energy. These channels bring life-giving nourishment through her blood to her cells and cleanse her body to carry illness away. If the channels are blocked, these critical functions will be impaired.

Children are more reactive to chemicals than adults because their carrying capacity for toxicity is much lower. And sensory kids in particular often have an even more deeply compromised ability to break down and clear those toxins. For children with weakened digestive and immune systems, even lower levels of toxicity will exceed that capacity and cause blocks to their energy channels. These harmful substances suppress health and put a tremendous burden on her system. So, while your child is struggling with sensory inputs that confuse and overwhelm her, she may be burdened by the additional effects of chemicals and toxins as well.

The Three Ways Toxins Enter the Body

There are three main ways toxins can enter a child's body. They can be ingested through foods, breathed in or absorbed through the skin.

My daughter was always hyper after she had candy or fruit roll-ups with red dye in it. She'd scream, tantrum and refuse to cooperate when she didn't get her way. I tried eliminating processed foods and was amazed at how quickly she calmed down and learned to handle not getting her own way all the time.

Mother of a 5-year-old

1. **Ingesting chemicals through foods.** It is very difficult to avoid chemicals in food. Even breast milk has toxins in it, albeit at very low levels. Fruits and vegetables are sprayed with chemicals, and processed foods are full of preservatives and dyes. Because there are many studies that point to red dyes as particularly troublesome, it is wise to get them completely out of your child's diet. Another challenge that has developed in recent years is the advent of laws that require that foods, served as snacks in schools and preschools, be only store-bought. Homemade snacks are not permitted. Unfortunately, most of the foods that end up being served to our children in these circumstances are highly processed and often dye-laden. And for a child with an immature sensory nervous system, the chemical burden is even higher. Here are some recommendations for *how to help reduce the toxic load* through ingestion:

   - **Buy organic** fruits and vegetables when you can.
   - **Become an avid label reader.** Watch out for food colorings, dyes and a long list of other chemicals. If there are any food colorings, especially red dye, in a food, do not buy it. The range of foods that contain red dye is surprising, but pay special attention to gelatin snacks, candy, beverages, ice creams, cheese and cookies. Don't be discouraged; there are plenty of popular brands that do not contain dyes. Be aware too, that some medicines (and even toothpastes!) contain dyes, so ask your doctor or pharmacist for alternatives.
   - **Cook from scratch** as much as possible to avoid the chemicals that enhance and preserve processed food.
   - **Take homemade snacks** to preschool (if your school allows) for your child so they can snack at the same time other children are having store-bought snacks.

2. **Breathing in chemicals.** Wouldn't it be nice if we could all spend our days near a high mountain lake, surrounded by air-purifying evergreens or at the beach breathing in clean air from the ocean? Of course, we all know that even these environments can be highly polluted in today's world, but you get the idea. We live in a world where harmful chemicals and other substances are unavoidably present in the air we breathe. Mercury is emitted from the garbage incinerator down the road and electric power plants that burn fossil fuels emit sulfur dioxide, carbon monoxide and a host of other unhealthy substances. The black, smoke-belching diesel truck in front of us at the stoplight signals to us that we are about to inhale something we'd prefer not to have in our lungs. We can't protect our children from all of this, nor are we suggesting that there is a specific, direct correlation between behavioral sensory problems and the presence of these substances in our world. But there are some inhaled chemicals that you can remove from your child's environment.

   The best tool a parent has for helping her child is her nose. If you can smell it, you might want to think about whether your child should be inhaling it. Do you, for example, really need air fresheners? Does your child react negatively on the days you clean your bathroom with various cleansers? There are good options available today for fragrance free and natural cleaning solutions. If your child pulls away when you are close, could it be your perfume or hair spray? Do you notice a reaction to the smell when she is playing with colored markers? Is there something in the air at a relative's house that seems to set your child off?

3. **Chemicals absorbed through the skin.** It is not easy to identify toxins that are absorbed by the skin, but as a parent, be on the lookout for possible triggers when your child experiences a sudden, otherwise unexplainable discomfort. Artificial fragrances are often the most likely to

trigger vulnerable and sensitive systems, and they are ubiquitous in products today. Perhaps the new clothes she is wearing have been somehow treated? Did you switch fabric softeners? (Do you need fabric softeners?) Is there scent in your detergent? Do you see a behavioral reaction after you've used a lotion on your child? Do you notice skin sensitivities to antibacterial sanitizers? You certainly shouldn't let your child's skin come into contact with cleaning products, even the mildest of them, except for mild soap and shampoo (with no artificial fragrances). You might even want to switch from deodorant soap to something milder.

One consistent source of skin (and inhalable) toxins for children are markers, including scented, washable and dry erase markers. To make them dry quickly, a solvent is often added that can make a child, even those without special challenges, become temporarily hyperactive. One of the parents in our study reported that her son got into markers one day and drew all over himself. He soon became distressed and lay on the couch rocking and moaning for what turned out to be days. When he returned to school, he couldn't remember his teachers' names. The parent reports that it was a month before he returned to his normal behavior. Although hyperactivity is the most common reaction, some children can become drowsy or 'out of it' after using them. It's a simple thing to switch to crayons and that is one of the first things you should do.

If you aren't certain about a chemical or potential toxin, remove it for a while, re-introduce it and watch for a reaction. New carpet, paint, paint thinner and construction adhesives can all create major reactions. And – and this is a hard one – don't forget to analyze what is happening at your child's day care, preschool or school. The industrial commercial cleaners and waxes used in some facilities leave long-lasting residue in the air. Ask questions, use your nose and look for patterns. This is not to suggest that you eliminate all the chemicals in your life that make things easier for you. You can't realistically go around policing every environment before you take your child there, but you can learn to become sensitive to your child's reactions in the presence of such chemicals.

All of this is clearly not going to be easy. Trying to pinpoint a reaction to one particular thing with a child who is reacting to several things all over the place takes a lot of energy. But remember, if you can eliminate an environmental cause of a troublesome behavior, you will save yourself and your child a tremendous amount of energy down the road and, most importantly, enhance your child's well-being and comfort. As you eliminate these toxins from your child's environment, you will find that your QST is working right along with you. The daily routine will help to reduce toxicity by opening the flow of energy and circulation so that, in many cases, her body can repair the damage on its own. Success will come in the form of those sticky, green, smelly poops that many children experience soon after beginning the QST program. It will tell you that the toxic load your child was carrying is leaving her body.

A Note on Food Allergies

My son has had a sensitive digestive system since the day he was born. My son is three and a half now and has been in the 'terrible twos' for about two years, which have been filled with lots of emotional meltdowns. He is really easily triggered into negative behavior. His motor development was pretty delayed. He would only walk a little bit, holding himself up on the wall and he wasn't very interested in playing. Once I took him off yogurt, eliminated the majority of cold foods and put him on cooked foods, within a short time, his chest was clearer and he had no nasal drainage. He's had a lot more energy and he started walking regularly on his own and started playing with his toys. The most amazing thing is that he stopped having the meltdowns. I feel more confident in his future now.

Mother of a 3 ½-year-old

It may seem odd to label some whole foods as toxic, but some children are unable to properly process certain kinds of food, even ones we normally consider healthy, creating an undigested load on the body that acts in ways similar to a man-made toxin. Controlled studies have shown that food allergies, especially those to milk and gluten, are fairly common in children. The substance in milk that we find troublesome is not lactose, as you might expect. It is casein. If your child is lactose intolerant, she will have the same kind of cramping and diarrhea after eating dairy products that so many in the general population experience. In the case of casein intolerance, it becomes a little harder to spot. Here are *five things that can indicate a gluten/casein food allergy*:

- **Voracious appetite.** Your child is constantly hungry for foods high in wheat or dairy, such as pizza. She might eat a huge amount of these foods and then exhibit anger when denied more. This is a sign that instead of creating a sense of fullness, the foods are triggering an unwanted chemical reaction in the body.
- **Desiring milk.** Your child wants to drink milk all day and the few foods she eats all contain milk or wheat. It is common for us to crave the very foods to which there is an allergy.
- **Aggression.** Your child becomes aggressive where she hadn't been before. This is often a side-effect of a drug, chemical or food that she cannot eliminate from her system.
- **Bloating.** The belly is bloated or tender to the touch. If your child won't lie on her belly, keep an eye out for other symptoms. A distended belly can be a response to a food allergy.
- **'Spacing out'.** Your child appears disconnected. Unprocessed chemicals from food allergies can knock us out just as those found in medicines can.

This is not to say that all children with sensory and behavioral problems should be on a gluten-free, casein-free diet (GFCF). Not all children have this intolerance. We have found that, if the intolerance is mild or moderate, an awareness of potential problems on the part of the parents results in a fairly natural reduction in troublesome foods. That often seems to be enough. This is because after a few months of QST, the child's appetite tends to open up, her digestive system works better and she begins to enjoy eating more. As she begins to try new foods, her diet comes into better balance and food intolerances disappear.

In the case of a severe intolerance, however, we have seen significant improvements after a child begins a GFCF diet. For example, we have had children in our research studies, initially not on gluten-free and dairy-free diets, who still made great strides improving sensory problems, constipation and sleep difficulties during the first two months with QST. But then they hit a plateau with no further progress in speech development and problems with aggression had not subsided. In many cases, we did see positive progress resume once parents switched to a GFCF diet at this point. There are several websites and books written about the GFCF diet if you are interested in giving it a try. It can be daunting at first because the typical American diet is filled with wheat and dairy, including cheese, yogurt, ice cream, bread, pasta and most snacks. It may be a little easier to think in terms of what your child *can* have: rice, potatoes, beans, rice milk, meat, fruit and lots of fresh cooked vegetables. For help on how to make this transition, start by checking with local parent support groups and branch out from there.

Importance of Rhythmic Daily Routines

We've talked about optimizing your child's diet so that she gets the energy and nutrients she needs. Now let's look at how to optimize her schedule and minimize her stress. Creating a balanced daily routine will provide opportunities for her to learn and grow every day as well as make sure that there is time for fun activities, family time, rest and relaxation. A routine allows you to pace your child's energy and minimize meltdowns that come from being tired or hungry.

Optimizing Your Child's Daily Energy Flow

Chinese medicine teaches us that children with developmental challenges have marked ebbs and flows in their daily energy cycle. It is a part of their physical functioning that simply has to be respected. When we go with a rhythmic flow of the day, children stay comfortable and learn better. When we go against it, children get stressed out. For most children with sensory and behavioral challenges (if digestion is working well), energy is stronger in the mornings, it dips after lunch and then rises again until dinner time. After dinner, it winds down until it is time for bed. That means that when your child wakes up in the morning, she is ready for the day. She has a certain amount of energy, but not enough to last the whole day. If she gets regular meals and alternates periods of activity with periods of rest, her batteries can recharge and last all day. That will be a day when she grows and learns comfortably. But for a sensory child, it takes even more energy to get through the day. They get tired sooner and the bottom falls out more rapidly. When they run out of gas, they get cranky, stubborn and can't deal with what is going on around them. So, let's think about how to make plans that are in tune with your child's changing energy levels throughout the day and sets a predictable and balanced daily routine.

One day, we were at the grocery store at about 2:00 in the afternoon and she had a full melt-down with crying, screaming and not being able to be consoled. I realized we had been going nonstop all day. I didn't fight, just left the groceries there, took her straight home and she fell immediately asleep for three hours.

Linda, mother of a 6-year-old

The Importance of Sleep

Sleep is an extremely important part of that daily routine. Just as awake time provides new experiences and the building blocks for growth, sleep provides the time and the space for that growth and restoration to happen. For all these reasons, good quality sleep is especially important for children with sensory and behavioral problems. Here are some of the benefits:

- The body relaxes completely and rests
- Emotional stress is discharged

- Energy reserves are recharged
- New things learned during the day are processed and integrated into memory
- Injuries are repaired
- Illnesses are treated
- The body and brain do most of their growing

Children usually start to establish a regular sleep cycle in their first year of life. They learn this by having a regular routine, regular naps and a regular bedtime. If your child has difficulty falling asleep or staying asleep, QST can be of great help. Once it becomes part of your bedtime routine, QST will help your child fall asleep and stay asleep all night.

Creating A Daily Routine

Let's go over the components of a daily routine that can be tuned to your child's energy. Here is what your child would need in her routine:

- Regular mealtimes to help to provide energy and nutrients
- A nap after lunch so she can digest her lunch and recharge her energy
- Alternating periods of activity with periods of quiet time (without technology)
- A bedtime routine to help her wind down for sleep
- A regular (and early) bedtime and a full night of undisturbed sleep

Regular meals are really important to keep the supply of energy and nutrients coming. And regular naps are important to pace your child's energy and prevent meltdowns. Naps give children a break before their energy hits bottom. In general, 1- and 2-year-olds will take two naps a day, and 5-year-olds will take one nap a day. The nap after lunch is especially important. It gives your child's body time to rest, digest and recharge right when her energy is running low. When she wakes up, she will have what she needs to get through the afternoon comfortably.

Plan your child's activities around her energy levels. She has energy for one period of activity in the morning and one in the afternoon. If she has preschool in the morning, make sure there is downtime after lunch. If there are family activities in the afternoon, make sure there is time to relax afterwards. Evenings are best for family time and winding down together. The bedtime routine starts her winding down, which leads to an easy transition into sleep. Bath, stories and cuddle time are helpful. And then off to bed at the same time every night. Aim for your child to be asleep by 8:00 pm and to sleep uninterrupted all night.

Table 12.1 Example: Daily routine for a 4-year-old

Time	Example for a 4-year-old
Wake- ups	7:00 AM
	cuddle time
Breakfast	8:00 AM
Activity	Pre-school, park, library
Lunch	12 noon
Nap	1–2 pm
Activity	Erands & appts with Mom, Play date
Down-time	Relaxation & playtime before dinner
Dinner	6:00pm
Activity	Family & playtime
Begin Bedtime Routine	7:30pm one-on-one with a parent
Asleep by	8:00 PM

Your Own Child's Daily Routine

To help you think about the patterns in your child's typical day, we've created the *Daily Routine Organizer* chart. The chart gives you spaces to fill in your child's activities for a week. There are no 'right answers' but by quickly jotting down each day's activities you will be able to see the structure of your child's actual daily routine. You can download and print out a copy from the QST Support Materials resource page at https://resourcecenter.routledge.com/books/9781032419299 (see access link in Appendix H, page 221) As you look at the chart, do you see any patterns in the weekly activities? Here are some questions that can help you think about optimizing her schedule:

1. Is there a time of day when your child is likely to have difficulties?
2. If so, could it be prevented with

   - a change in the routine;
   - a nap;
   - a meal; or
   - quiet time?

3. Does your child have a regular (and early) bedtime?
4. Does your child start and end her day with cuddle time with a parent?

In Conclusion

When you combine QST with your attention to diet, nutrition, sleep and a focus on the healing effects of rhythm and structure in daily life, you now have a number of powerful tools that you can use at home to provide your sensory child with all she needs to grow into a healthy, independent and loving adult.

Part III

Guiding Your Way With 52 Weekly Letters

Introduction to Weekly Letters

Our goal is to make this a successful year of QST for you and your child. Because improvements are cumulative and positive changes are built on your repetition of the QST movements each day, we plan to be there with you, week by week, to help you maintain that consistency. To do that, we've created this year-long series of weekly letters to guide, encourage and support you along the way. For each week, you will find a personal letter waiting for you. Every letter is short, from one to a few pages, and designed to take just a few minutes out of your busy day. We've written each to address the kinds of questions that we know come up for parents at each step of the process. Mostly written by the two of us – Louisa and Linda – some letters are from our QST Master Trainers and others from parents who share their own helpful tips and experiences.

We've organized the 52 letters into seven sections, each relating to a common theme. Our first section focuses on learning the basics of the daily routine in the beginning weeks, including your own self-care. We show you what signs of progress and distress to look for and how best to adapt your touch technique to respond to resistances and open up roadblocks. As the weeks progress and you feel more comfortable with the basics, our next section of letters addresses how to use the daily routine to relieve and support common problems with regulation including sleep, listening, tantrums and emotional regulation. We know the times when you may need a little help to stay consistent. That's when our letters focus on the 'dog days' and how to successfully navigate through them. This will bring us to mid-year, where we will guide you through completing a second set of parent checklists and a mid-year progress chart so you can see the progress you've already made and re-focus your goals for the months ahead.

As you move into the second half of the year, we offer some extra techniques and talk more deeply about how QST works to address some common issues like dealing with transitions, emotional bubbles and enlisting other family members to help with the daily routine. As you reach the end of the year, we will focus on more specific needs including addressing regressions, certain developmental or medical conditions and the lifelong importance of early self-regulation. At year's end, we'll help you take stock of your progress and offer some final thoughts for the future.

Getting the Most Out of the Weekly Letters

Over the years we've come to know what types of questions come up for parents and at what points in the year, so we've intentionally written these letters in a sequence that matches the experience of many children and parents that have gone before you. However, you can also use the

DOI: 10.4324/9781003360421-17

table of contents for the weekly letters as a reference guide to jump ahead whenever a problem area arises. By scanning the letters by title, you can quickly look up and get help with a specific concern at any point. For example, if your child is reacting to stressful situations with biting, kicking, pinching or hitting, scan through the list to find "*A simple technique to stop aggressive behaviors*" in Week 33. Or, if you observe your child reacting to your touch with either pain or ticklishness, jump to Weekly Letter 7, which focuses on that particular issue.

We've also purposefully organized the letters into thematic groupings so you can use them as a general reference guide whenever you need help to work through specific sensory, behavioral or developmental difficulties as they arise. For example, the **Extra Techniques** section includes letters that will help you when your child is having difficulties with transitions. Other letters in the grouping provide you with helpful techniques when you child is highly agitated or defensive. And our group of letters labeled **QST for Specific Needs** will help you through regressions and also provide you with a new way to look at developmental phases such as "*Stuck in stress mode*" (Week 43), which used to be (mis)labeled as 'the terrible twos', or "*Reframing the need for control*" (Week 44), (mis)labeled in previous years as 'the controlling fours'. We've also created an extensive index at the back of the book to make it easier to find answers to particular questions or difficulties.

Fifty-two weeks may seem like a long time, but our autism research has clearly shown that progress continues to grow through the year for parents who are consistent with the daily routine. We want to support you at each step along the way so you too can see these benefits.

Parents sometimes ask why it takes that much time – it's because your child's sensory system may have been out of kilter for some years. When that happens, her brain and body follow their own particular patterns of growth and development. And when a body or a brain 'gets stuck' in such a pattern, it takes time, repetitive effort and energy to change and forge more healthy pathways.

Think of yourself as being more like a good gardener than an auto mechanic. It might be nice if we could 'fix things', like changing out a broken part, but bringing more organized patterns to your child's nervous system and encouraging renewed development isn't a mechanical process. We're working with a living, dynamic system, and living systems have their own pace and timing. The repetition of new and healthier patterns is what you are offering with the regularity of QST. You are helping to change old patterns and replace them with new, more integrated and regulated ones. You are helping your child improve the way *she takes in sensory information, how she learns* and *how she relates to others*. All of this takes time.

Mastering the Basics – Weeks 1–14

Week 1

Patting or Pressing – Learning What Works Best

Dear parents,

✓ OK! You've read the book and watched the online videos.

✓ You've practiced the routine and feel reasonably comfortable with the 12 movements.

✓ You've filled out the *Sensory and Self-Regulation Checklist* and the *Parenting Stress Index* at the end of Chapter 7. These will give you a beginning record to track your progress in the months ahead.

✓ You have the *QST Sensory Movements Chart* [from Appendix A] handy so you can refer to it, and you're ready to begin the daily QST routine with your child.

While each of these is important steps to getting started, the most important part of QST is how you learn to observe and adapt your touch to your child's responses. QST is not just a 12-step 'recipe' or a one-size-fits-all treatment. How you attune your touch to make it comfortable and relaxing for your child is what makes QST unique and so effective.

For your first week, you'll have to figure out what kind of touch your child responds to best for each of the movements, patting or pressing. How will you know? It's not hard. You are already tuned in to your child and you know best what he likes and what he doesn't like. Just follow those cues to find which touch technique he responds most positively to. Older children or children with good verbal skills will also be able to tell you what feels best. Encourage them to let you know.

Pressing. Most children with sensory difficulties tend to be over-sensitive and respond best to pressing, especially the slow deep pressing movements. In fact, the first three QST movements generally start with slower, deeper pressing down the arms, then on the chest and then the belly. As you continue through the rest of the movements, you'll need to choose between patting and pressing. Even if you can only do pressing at the start, in time you'll be able to switch to some patting movements, a shift that will signal a big first step in normalizing a sensory child's over-sensitivity to touch. For over-sensitivity, pressing improves tolerance to touch because it by-passes the highly sensitive nerve endings at the surface of the skin, engages the touch receptors deep in the muscles and turns on the relaxation response.

DOI: 10.4324/9781003360421-18

Patting. However, if your child is more on the under-sensitive side, you will need to use patting to get him to register the sensations. Patting opens up his awareness of the skin and his connection to that body part. Under-sensitive children usually need to start with a lot of patting on the top of head and back of the body (in the 'down the back' and 'down the back – two hands' movements – see Chapter 8, Movements 5 and 6) to open up awareness. One good sign that your child has begun to open up to sensations is when he starts to hum while you pat. Humming is a cue that you've found an area that needs more touch. Be sure to pat a little longer on those areas where he starts humming. Once he allows you to switch to some pressing movements, that will signal that he is beginning to feel the different parts of his body come together as a whole.

The goal is to find the combination of patting or pressing that allows your child to tolerate each of the movements in a quiet and relaxed way. Don't worry if you don't understand it all at first. It's a lot to grasp in the beginning and you just need to do the best you can each day. Over time, you'll find these skills will come quite naturally.

Our very best wishes for your journey,

Louisa and Linda

Week 2

Parent Self-Care and Self-Compassion

Dear parents,

It's natural for a parent to be concerned for the physical comfort and well-being of their child and to forgive them when they've made a mistake. But it's not always easy for parents to do that for themselves. That's why this week, we're asking you to think as much about your own physical comfort as you do about your child's and to be as forgiving of yourself as you are of them.

Finding a Comfortable Position

Your child will feel calm and safe when you are. However, for you to feel calm and relaxed, you must first get comfortable. So, to set yourself up for success from the beginning, it is important to find a position to give QST in a way that protects your own body and comfort. If you are either unaware that you are uncomfortable or push through any discomfort you might feel, chances are you will find reasons to stop QST prematurely and not really know why. We encourage you to truly think as much about yourself and your own physical comfort as you do about your child's. Are you in a place and a position where you are comfortable and not putting strain on your body, a position that allows you to be relaxed and comfortable? Here are some important tips to protect your back.

- **Keep your child close.** To maintain your own comfort and balance, it is best to keep your child close to you. We've found it is often difficult for parents to protect their own backs while doing QST on their child's bed. If you do find this to be the best place, be sure to move your child next to the edge of the bed, close to you, and ensure that you don't have to reach to the middle.

- **On the floor.** Some parents use a favorite blanket or quilt and find a comfortable place sitting on the floor. Here, again, make sure your position doesn't put undue strain on your back or knees.
- **Sofas and ottomans.** Other parents will kneel next to the sofa, ottoman or hassock. If your child fits on an ottoman or hassock, pull it out so you have access to both sides of your child. Experiment with ways to kneel or sit comfortably next to your child as you do the routine.
- **Using a table.** Some parents chose to buy a portable massage table online or use a thick blanket or pad on a sturdy table at home. If you are standing, keep the height of the area you have your child on at about your waist level. *Make sure you can protect your child from a fall if they move fast!*
- **Above all,** experiment with different places and different heights until you find the spot comfortable for *you* and your child.

Self-Compassion – What if I Make Mistakes?

Parents are often afraid of making mistakes. But it's normal to feel uncertain when you are learning something new. With QST, the big mis-steps are obvious and easy to avoid: ignoring your child's body cues or giving the treatment when you are sick, angry or upset. Feel assured, if you follow the Qigong movements downwards from the head toward the hands and feet and always *follow your child's cues*, you won't harm your child. And making mistakes is part of the learning process! When you make a mistake, forgive yourself, and if it was significant or upsetting, ask forgiveness from your child. How you repair the moment is more important than any mistake you make. As you do the treatment every day, the touch techniques will become second nature and your skills at reading your child's body language will get better and better. Soon your child will start asking you for QST.

Take care,
Linda and Louisa

Week 3

Getting Started

Lessons From a Mother

A letter to you fellow warriors,

I first learned about QST from two other mothers. It was the only therapy in their list of suggestions that I hadn't tried yet. I had already tried even more therapies than the ones on their list. Checking on the QSTI website, out of the various ways to learn, I opted for the less time-consuming and more affordable solution, to buy the books and learn at home. "What is the worst-case scenario?", I thought, "I spend some money for books, which if not useful, I could always donate to the library?"

Waiting for the books to be delivered, I contacted a very knowledgeable certified QST instructor I also found on the website, who navigated me through the books and made herself available for questions. Suddenly, I wasn't alone; I had somebody to share and to guide me through the experience. Once the books arrived, as you can guess, I became overwhelmed as I started to read. A week had already passed, I hadn't finished the book and I hadn't started the QST routine with my son. I felt like I had started losing motivation, so one evening I opened the book, put my child on the couch and just started.

My first mistake was that I wanted to finish the 12 movements all at once. I did it, but my child was upset, cried and pulled my hair. I went to my notebook and I wrote under Day 1, "At least I had started." The next afternoon, he had, to my surprise, dark green stools without having eaten a dark green food. Imagine my surprise when I saw that as one of the described reactions after day one. So, I decided that this 'procedure' – because at that time it was a 'procedure' and not a shared activity as it is supposed to be – had to be done daily.

I had the diagrams with me before and during every session, even if my child was throwing it away or was trying to tear it. I had to go through a lot of hair pulling, crying and pushing. A week later, I downloaded the video made by Dr. Silva herself. I should have done that before starting to read the books. I saw how gentle, patient and confident she was, not to mention that I realized that I had performed some parts of the QST routine 100% wrong! The video gave me a new perspective and I continued more motivated.

Two weeks after we started the sessions, my son's physical therapist noticed differences and asked me what I did differently. Also, I noticed the total absence of potty accidents during the day. Two-and-half months later, we had a long session with a certified QST therapist. The same afternoon, my son attended a two-hour class and his diaper stayed dry during the whole night. And then COVID-19 came. My son ceased all his activities and started having accidents, along with behaviors of frustration. We had accidents all through March, but in April he started having eye contact again during the QST and a little better bladder control. I was ready to quit, but our therapist was there for me to give support and to help me continue.

QST is very unique and different from all other therapies. Why?

1. It can have very positive results, different for everybody and at a different pace, but it does!
2. It starts as a therapy, but it becomes a daily activity. It is shared by the whole family, since the daily routine can be given by different members of the family and even by two members who help and complement each other.
3. It is flexible and grows with you. It can be done at different times of the day, as many times as you want, in bed, on the floor, on the couch, with or without the iPad, cell phone etc.; you can skip days if exhausted or sick, and you can adapt your touch to suit your child's needs.
4. It doesn't matter if you make mistakes. (I make mistakes every day and I've been doing it for six months.)
5. It is a bonding experience because it reflects the battles of parents and children and their victories.

If our therapist wasn't a one-and-a-half-hour drive one way, I would ask her to give him a session once a week because I noticed so much progress from the one session we had with her.

Maria, mother of super explosive 10-year-old.

Week 4

Working With Resistance to Touch

When we started QST, we found it pretty difficult for a few weeks. Our son would resist the movements, push me away and complain that his body hurt. But pretty soon he started to enjoy the treatment. Then the changes started – he slept and ate better, played on his own and his language got a lot clearer. It was so worth sticking with it through those first hard weeks.

Mother of a 3-year-old

Dear parents,

It is quite common for children to resist or refuse the QST movements in the beginning when the sensations are unfamiliar and can easily trigger a fight-flight reaction. We know that this refusal can feel very unsettling to even the most conscientious parent and disturb your own all-important ability to remain calm. So, at this stage, it's important that you don't force any of the movements or get into a struggle by insisting on completing them. That will only make things worse and undermine the real goal, which is a calm and relaxed connection. First, chose the quietest time in your child's day, when he isn't too tired or too hungry, as both conditions can increase already heightened sensitivities.

The following suggestions will help to make it easier for your child to tolerate the movements until the daily routine improves his response to touch and he comes to enjoy and even ask for it. For example, some children will resist completely at first, while others can tolerate the first few minutes of the routine but then become overwhelmed, distracted or insist on stopping. If your child resists or becomes overwhelmed, don't be afraid to take a short (cuddle) break, maybe one or two minutes at most, then try to go back and pick up where you left off. Don't let these breaks get so long that your child gets involved in some other activity. Short breaks often help children to accept the protocol for longer and longer periods and you will find that his resistance will disappear in a few weeks.

Still, we know that these first few weeks can be very difficult and that taking breaks does not always do the trick. The QST routine calls for you to start with your child lying down but not all children are ready to do that. If necessary, it's okay to start with your child either standing or sitting. Do the movements the best you can, where you can. At this stage, don't get too worried about doing things perfectly, you have to start where your child is. If two adults are available, it's helpful for one parent to gently and comfortably hold your child in their lap with your child facing out (your child's back snuggled up against the parent's chest). Most importantly, *do not restrain your child!* This will only heighten the fight-flight response and cause him to struggle. With both adults 'lending' their calm, this gently encompassing hold will often provide a sense of safety and make it easier for the other parent to begin the movements.

She still resists some, but is getting a little calmer during the routine. She can tolerate Movements 1 and 2 now and sometimes Movements 3 and 4 before we have to take a little break. So that's progress!

Father of a 4-year-old

But we know that even *that* may not always succeed. In today's distractible times, only TV or a video can occupy some children's attention. Using videos is not ideal, but if you find that this is the *only* way to get started, that is perfectly okay too. Get your child involved in his favorite video while you calmly sit next to him and begin some of the basic movements. Some of the movements call for eye contact. Don't worry about that at this stage, that will come later. For now, your intention is to get through as many of the steps as you can to help your child begin to experience touch with greater comfort and to be able to hold eye contact with you.

It may take several weeks or in some cases even a few months, but try to wean your child slowly away from the videos because they are inherently stimulating to the nervous system – just the opposite of what we are trying to do! If, for example, you start with him watching a video on your phone, watch to see when his eyes leave the screen and then slowly turn the phone over. When he wants it back, turn it back for him. You will notice that over time, his attention will increasingly wander away from the video. We have found that eventually, even the most resistant child can learn to do without this distraction. In time, as his use of video decreases, begin to focus more on making direct eye contact.

Most importantly, don't give up! Resistance is only a phase, and your child will definitely pass through it. Keep up the good work! Your child's enjoyment of touch really will improve and QST can become a special time together.

Warmest wishes,

Louisa and Linda

Week 5

Lending Your Calm

Dear parents,

You'll find that your own emotions make up a very important part of your attuned touch. That's because while your child is responding to *what* you are doing, he is even more tuned in to your feelings *while* you are doing it. The profound love and commitment you feel for your child is what makes this parent-provided intervention so effective. When you are relaxed and focused on your child during the movements your calm, loving energy is transmitted through your touch, your voice and your reassuring presence. The QST movements are designed to make the most of this heart-to-heart connection. And it's through that connection that you are 'loaning' him the feelings of calm and safety until he can learn from you what that experience is all about and how he can do it for himself through self-regulation.

With all that you do for everyone in your family we know how difficult it is to find that place of calm for yourself. The following simple exercise can help. Focusing on your breath can be one of the best ways to release your own stress and find that loving place within yourself to connect to your child and begin QST each day.

- Start by standing quietly and connecting to your body by feeling your feet flat on the floor. Then rub your hands together to feel the warmth and loving energy that you will use in your touch.
- Close your eyes for a moment and take a slow deep in-breath.

- Let your shoulders drop down and allow the relaxation to wash over you as you make a long, slow exhale.
- Repeat for 2–3 breaths, focusing especially on the exhale until you feel centered, connected and ready to begin.

Neuroscience research shows that when you exhale, your brain sends a signal that slows the heart and turns on your own rest-relax-relate response. By gently focusing on and extending your exhale you can deepen the relaxation response both for yourself and for your child. With practice, a deeper in-breath will come about effortlessly.

You can use this exercise to center yourself before you begin the QST routine. It's also a helpful tool to re-center yourself if you find you are tensing with frustration if your child resists a particular QST movement and pushes you away. You can also use this exercise anytime throughout the day to calm and center yourself, especially at times when your child's meltdown pulls you into his revved-up reaction state or when you are simply having to rush too quickly through your day. Stop for just a moment, feel your feet on the ground, then take a slow deep in-breath and focus on a slow, deep out-breath.

Peaceful wishes,

Louisa and Linda

Week 6

Attuning to Your Child's Energy Level to Bring Calm

Dear parents,

QST focuses on attunement to touch that is reciprocal, which means that it allows for an instantaneous back-and-forth non-verbal communication that is often more powerful than words. But we sometimes forget about another important form of connection – energy – which is also reciprocal and can even be contagious. Children with sensory challenges are often highly energetic and 'on the go', which makes it difficult to begin the QST treatment. When this happens, parents often become tense and agitated, elevating their own energy and rushing through the routine. We want to share Danny's story, taken from Orit Tal-Atzili's early intervention QST program, to illustrate how parents can attune to and meet their child's energy level with the same awareness they used to attune their touch. You'll see how Danny's mother's attunement supported her daily QST during the challenging first weeks, and how she was able to bring Danny's energy down.

Danny started QST after receiving early intervention services for about a year without making much progress. As a baby, he was irritable and difficult to soothe. Referred to the QST program at 28 months, Danny's parents were very frustrated with his challenging behaviors, including aggression and non-compliance, running off in unsafe ways and hour-long meltdowns. While Danny was very communicative non-verbally, he was not yet saying any words, was a picky eater and would not sit down to eat. He had no purposeful play with toys and was constantly seeking attention and sensory stimulation (crashing into things, jumping, running, rough housing, throwing, hitting his sister and his pets, etc.). He insisted on sleeping with his parents, who needed to hold him down for over an hour in order for him to fall asleep. He constantly moved in his sleep, so his parents did not get much sleep either. Danny was also over-sensitive to touch and resisted all care activities. His parents had to forcefully restrain him in order to brush his teeth. Given Danny's high energy level, constant motion, sensitivities and agitation, one can easily imagine how challenging it was to start and then to complete the daily QST routine with him.

For the first two weeks of QST, Danny kept wiggling out and running away. Even when his family worked together (parents and grandma were trained), they were unable to finish all the QST movements at one sitting. What helped us move forward was Danny's mother's attunement to his energy needs and how she intuitively developed a variety of effective responses and distractions that gradually allowed her to complete the treatment. When she invariably had to stop before completion, she always returned to the routine later that day, when his energy level was more accessible (she continued from where she had stopped). To distract him from his disruptive activity, she patiently gave Danny family photos and told him little stories about them while she quietly resumed the treatment. When necessary, she would follow him around the house while still tapping and/or use the TV tuned to a calm show on low volume (e.g., children's lullabies).

QST is all about attuning to your child's responses, never forcing the movement but constantly observing to make sure the technique is not triggering or escalating your child's stress response. The goal is to always adapt the technique to a calming and organizing form of touch that your child accepts and calms down with. Danny's mother instinctively did all this. Using creative methods, she attuned to his overwhelming energy level. She did not confront him. She adjusted and redirected to offer more organizing activities that helped Danny to calm down. She refrained from corrective verbal instructions. Instead, she 'spoke' to him in his own non-verbal language using her touch rather than her words to communicate with Danny's energy. To ensure that her own energy matched what Danny needed, she worked hard on herself to remain calm, positive, and supportive.

In these early weeks when QST was still so challenging, what kept Danny's parents going was faith in the process, as well as noticing positive changes, including decreased aggression and better sleep, attention and compliance. By five months, Danny was combining two or three words together with clearer articulation. He started to sleep through the night in his own bed, helped with little chores and showed empathy to others and kindness toward his little sister. No more diapers! No more bottles! No more cruelty to animals! Danny's parents stated that he became a "completely different child" and that "many of our behavioral issues have disappeared". They continued QST for about one year, then stopped when they had no more sensory concerns. By then it took them about 10 minutes each day to do his QST. About a year after stopping QST, Danny's mother sent this update:

QST helped Danny through his sensory issues. We are now able to breeze through basic grooming in the morning and night. He has learned coping and ways to calm his emotions. He is also a much better eater and transitions from one activity to the next pretty seamlessly . . . QST has been invaluable to us, life changing and the best thing I believe I could have ever done for Danny and our family!

If you notice that your child's energy is skyrocketing and it's hard to start the QST routine, you can follow Danny's mother's example. Stay calm and positive, respect your child's cues and allow them some choices and control. Engage in a quiet and meaningful activity (like Danny's family pictures) and let them show you where they want to be. Instead of positioning them, with your own sense of calm, follow them around and get back to the treatment as soon as they stop moving, wherever that may be (and even if they are still standing). Be aware and attuned to your child's energy *and* bring your own energy down. Danny's mother did this by creating a feeling of comfort and safety that allowed him to accept the QST routine. By being positive, aware, patient, calm and open minded, you can do this too!

Best wishes,

Orit and Linda

Orit Tal-Atzili, OTD, OTR/L

Certified QST Trainer and Master Trainer

Rockville, Maryland, USA

www.qsti.org/meet-our-master-trainers.html

To read more about Dr. Tal-Atzili's program, see Appendix F – QST in Early Intervention.

Week 7

Pain and Ticklishness

Dear parents,

Pain and ticklishness are two of the most common causes of resistance to parent touch in the early weeks of QST. These sensations are triggered when certain areas of your child's skin aren't processing touch signals normally and, in turn, lead to resistance in the form of a fight-or-flight response. While it is natural for parents to avoid uncomfortable areas, the signs of painfulness or ticklishness are telling us exactly *where* the key locations are that need our special attention in the daily routine. The body areas where things are uncomfortable and/or painful for your child provides you with a *very important clue*! Giving those uncomfortable areas skillful attention is important because those sensitivities are often at the root of behavioral problems and can create roadblocks to progress when they are avoided. To help normalize touch sensations and the behaviors that they cause, we feel it is very important to re-visit how to work with these uncomfortable areas. This week, let's take a look at the discomfort of pain and ticklishness, two common problems for children, and what you can do to help.

Pain. When your child is experiencing discomfort or pain, he will wince, pull away from you or try to push your hands away. For children with over-reactive sensory systems, even the most loving touch can actually feel painful. It's quite natural for parents to stop and avoid these areas, but pain is a signal that tells you that you've found a place that needs your skilled touch the most. It's important at these times to *adapt your touch technique* to the type of touch that your child can tolerate so you can continue and help that area to normalize its sensory signals to the brain and feel better! The most common areas where you will find pain reactions are around the ears, base of the skull, on the fingers and especially on toes. Other areas may show up as well (chest, tummy). **What to do to fix it:** If you find an area of pain or discomfort, don't stop! Don't move away from it. Just switch to the opposite technique. So, if you had been patting, switch to slower pressing, and if you were pressing, then switch to patting. Watch to see if your child begins to relax; that is the sign that you can continue with the rest of the protocol. If there is still a pain reaction, don't pull away. Stop the movement and rest the warmth and weight of your hands quietly on the area that is painful. Calmly, gently say, "You're okay, Mommy [Daddy, etc.] will make it feel better." This gives your child a moment to quiet the fight-or-flight response. Then you can try again with the slower, deeper pressing movements. For fingers or toes, you can encircle and hold the painful finger(s) or toe(s) between the warmth of your palms and gently start to apply a slow, pulsing pressure. Fingers can take a month or longer to get better and ears can take longer, especially for children who suffer from severe speech delays. Toes often take the longest, sometimes several months.

Ticklishness. Ticklishness and giggling are signs that the skin is often over-sensitive. A common sign that your child is ticklish is, of course, giggling, but cringing and pulling away can also be a sign. The neck, fingers, toes, tummy, sides of chest or legs can all feel ticklish. If you see your child hunching his shoulders and pulling away, that is often a sign that the neck is ticklish.
What to do to fix it: When your child shows ticklishness in a certain area, try to stay on that area, but slow down and switch to slower, deeper pressing. Continue this for a while and the giggling and discomfort should stop. Remember to look for this sign the next time your do the routine. The ticklishness will often be gone in a few days.

Pain and ticklishness are the most common problems to overcome because the majority of children tend to be over-sensitive. In fact, whether over- or under-sensitive, QST is specifically designed to integrate touch signals to the brain and make your child more comfortable in his skin. As that happens, you'll find that his resistance will melt away. Next week we'll look at the most common problem with under-sensitivity – numbness.

All our best,
Louisa and Linda

Week 8

Numbness

Dear parents,
Not every child has numbness, but for those who do, it is important to know how to work with it in your daily routine. You can't actually see numbness. You will only see the signs indirectly when your child doesn't register your touch or when your child hurts himself but doesn't cry. Or, you may not even know there has been numbness because he calmly allows you to do the treatment for weeks, but then suddenly responds as if it hurts or as if he's afraid and starts pushing you away when you get to those areas. We've seen this happen in many of the children we have worked with. As the numbness improves, the skin begins to feel again, and he can shift from an under-reactive to an over-reactive phase as he starts to register unfamiliar sensations and those areas begin to feel uncomfortably over-stimulated for a short time.

This new burst of sensitivity is a sign of real improvement and marks a very important transition point. It means that your skilled touch has helped bring feeling into these areas and allowed him to be more aware of his body. Your child will need time and your support to adjust to all of these new sensations, and you can help him do this when you recognize this as a new phase and attune your touch to meet it.

What to do to fix it: As with pain and ticklishness, the first thing to do is to immediately switch all of your movements to pressing. Don't move the skin much – just press gently and rhythmically in that area. When you move to the next area, don't slide your hands over his skin (sliding on the skin is more stimulating). Pick your hands up and move to the next spot before beginning the rhythmic pressing again. Deeper pressing at this point will increase your child's tolerance to touch and calm his nervous system. Within a few weeks, this uncomfortable phase will pass, touch will begin to feel good and the numbness will subside. As this happens, he will begin to feel normal pain when injured and enjoy being cuddlier and more affectionate. Importantly, when your child can begin to feel pain and pleasure, he will open up to new feelings in his own body. That is the beginning of real empathy because once he is open to feeling his own body, he can be open to the feelings of others. What wonderful rewards for making it through the hyper-sensitivity phase!

He said he felt a cut on his thumb and asked for a band aid! This was new.

Father of a 2 ½-year-old

He feels his hands when they are cold now and will wear his mittens.

Mother of a 4-year-old

She can feel pain now. She's also stopped biting me and actively hugs me. Qigong works!

Mother of a 5-year-old

While we have described over-sensitive areas (painful or ticklish) and under-sensitive areas (numbness) as being separate, children often experience a mix of both. In the coming weeks, watch for each of these signs, quite possibly in different areas of your child's body, and adapt your technique to each area. Don't avoid the over- or under-sensitive places. Your patient and consistent focus on these problem areas will open your child's blockages to touch and allow for healthy development to resume.

Keep up the good work!

Louisa and Linda

Week 9

Signs QST is Working

Dear parents,

Every square inch of our skin is connected to our brains by millions of tiny sensory nerves that create a vast network of 'skin-brain connections'. These circuits play a crucial role in helping the brain to grow and learn. But when these connections are dormant or not well integrated, it leads to sensory difficulties. As you help your child's skin feel better with QST, you also help to strengthen and integrate this sensory network. Some signs that you are waking up or activating these circuits may seem very obvious to you, while for others, you will have to watch more closely. Let's take a look at the signs of these new skin-brain connections so you can recognize and support them as they are taking place:

Signs that he relaxes to touch:

You see these signs beginning with the first two pressing movements as you move down the arms and relax the chest:

- He stops struggling with touch and the QST routine.
- He lies down when the treatment starts.
- He lays his head down while on his tummy (movement down back).
- He relaxes his body.

These signs also unfold in progressive stages as you do the movements down the head, neck and back.

Signs that he connects with you and his own body:

- **Humming** shows he is connecting with his body and enjoying your touch. When this happens, be sure to stay right where you are when the humming starts. Keep the same pressure and rhythm right on that spot and don't go on to the next movement until the humming stops. Children may often hum as you pat down their backs.
- **Making eye contact** is a very good sign and signals that he is making a connection with you. You will often get eye contact when you are working on the arms and hands and when you get a relaxation response while working on his chest.
- **Smiling at you** signals he is communicating his pleasure and connection.

Signs that he's finding ways to self-soothe:

Self-soothing is the gold standard for the QST technique. When this happens, it signals the beginning of the most important goal of all: self-regulation and the ability for deep relaxation. You may see these early signs of self-soothing while you are working on relaxing the chest:

- Closing the eyes
- Rubbing the eyes
- Yawning

These three signs can occur at any point in your treatment. While easy to spot, all of them (humming, rubbing the eyes, yawning) are easy to overlook. When giving QST, these are not seen as random movements. They are clear signals that you are on the right track and that important progress has begun. Take notice and pleasure in your accomplishment!

Great work!

Louisa and Linda

Week 10

More Signs QST is Working

Dear parents,

Last week, we covered some of the more obvious signs that you are making good progress with QST (humming, rubbing eyes and yawning). This week, we'd like to remind you of some of the signs that, while not so obvious and easier to overlook, are equally important signals that you are activating the skin-brain connections. Signs that brain activity is taking place are of course very hard to pin down or identify. But it is very important that you be alert to these not-so-obvious signs because while they involve very small movements that most of us would overlook or see as just random, they can signal big and positive shifts in the touch-brain connection. We have identified two very specific body cues and behaviors that, when they occur, signal these changes at work. Here's what to look that indicate parts of his brain that may have been "asleep" are activated and integrating:

- **Spontaneous movements of the lips and tongue** when working on the fingers. Your child may make little pursing movements of his lips, or his tongue may explore the inside of his cheeks. For children with more serious speech difficulties, we have found that these movements can be an early sign of improved vocalization, indicating that the touch-brain connection in this particular area has been activated. If you see these spontaneous movements of the lips and tongue, particularly in a child with speech difficulties, pay special attention and be sure to stay a little longer with more repetitions of that movement. For children who have been picky eaters, these movements often precede a new openness to trying different foods and textures.
- **Small twitching or fluttering movements of the eyes and face** often happen toward the end of the very last step, Movement 12 (nourish and integrate). These signal that the brain is making connections and that your child has begun to integrate all the sensory information that your touch and intention has conveyed throughout the whole routine. When you see these signs, and especially when your child is also deeply relaxed, do additional repetitions of this movement to quietly finish.

Watch carefully for all of these small and easy-to-miss signals. They are important because they tell you that your use of the QST is beginning to really impact the skin-brain connection while building the three skills necessary for growth and development: how to relax, how to connect socially and how to stay calm and feel good in the presence of another person. You should feel very proud and happy when you see any of these signs. They signal the beginnings of self-regulation and improved social skills.

This is good work you're doing.

All our best,

Louisa and Linda

Week 11

Opening Roadblocks to Development

Dear parents,

Now that you've been doing QST for several weeks, we hope the daily routine has started to become second nature to you. We also hope that you've been able to identify and begin to work through those areas that may be uncomfortable for your child. Staying with the areas of discomfort and helping your child work through them does much more than you might think. Over- or under-sensitivity to touch has often interfered or prevented children from achieving some basic steps in development (see Chapter 2 – Self-Regulation – A Parent's Gift). So, when you work on uncomfortable areas, you help not only to wake up numb areas or calm down painful or ticklish areas but also to open up old roadblocks to development that those sensory difficulties created in the first place. For example, when the sensations of touch are normalized on the sides the spine during the 'down the back' in Movement 5, children start to feel the sensation of needing to go to the bathroom and now feel the wetness of their diaper. That's when potty training gets much easier and more spontaneous.

Similar changes occur when sensitivity in the fingers is normalized. One of the very first steps for early communication, called gestural language, involves the simple ability for a child to point to what he wants. For some children, such basic gestural language may never get out of the starting gate. That's because they don't have an integrated sense of feeling or awareness of their fingers. So, it is important to work on the sensitivity of the fingers until they feel comfortable. Once you bring normal feeling into the fingers, your child can begin to use them to point. This is especially important for the very young. As you normalize touch in the fingers, it helps to create a direct connection between the fingers and the speech area of the brain. For children under the age of six, this process often takes a month or less.

For children with more severe problems, we have often found that normalizing touch sensitivity in the fingers can help the lips and the tongue to awaken to the sensations necessary for speech and for tolerating food textures. When this happens, it can mean that you have activated those connections to the brain and have helped to jump-start speech. And for all children, even those who already have language, proper sensations in the fingers are necessary for important fine motor skills.

Reducing your child's sensitivity to touch can also help support several other basic skills. Take listening, for example. The child whose skin feels uncomfortable will naturally avoid everything that has to do with his ears and will avoid all touch in that area. When you adapt your touch in Movements 7 and 8 you help him to tolerate those feelings and begin to normalize the feeling around the ears (by either reducing over- or under-sensitivity). This allows your child to move out of fight-flight-or-freeze mode so the muscles of the inner ear can relax and his hearing can improve. He can start to use his ears and be more responsive and attentive to you, his teachers and his friends.

So, when you reduce your child's discomfort to touch, you bring more than just moments of calm to his nervous system. You create new, more organized sensory pathways for social, emotional and mental growth to resume. Helping your child work through his sensory difficulties connects to many important areas, including sleep, speech, attention, social connection and all forms of self-regulation. It's all inter-connected. As you normalize your child's ability to experience pleasurable touch, you help open the doorway to your child's healthy development.

Good work! And best wishes,

Louisa and Linda

Week 12

Persisting Through Frustrating and Difficult Times

Reflections From a QST Master Trainer

Note: In Dr. Tal-Atzili's letter below, we have **bolded** and *italicized* sections to highlight for you specific adaptations to both touch and technique that she used to address initial resistance and over-sensitive reactions. These adaptations demonstrate how you can adapt your own technique to address issues specific to your child.

Dear Parents,

I have worked with children as an occupational therapist (OT) for over 25 years, but it wasn't until I became familiar with QST that I found an intervention that consistently made significant differences in regulating a child's sensory system. I want to share the following story of a child with intensive sensory and regulation needs. I hope the struggles, as well as the successes that followed, will inspire you to continue giving your child the daily QST even through the frustrating or difficult times.

Adrian's story

Adrian was referred to QST when he was almost three years old because he had not achieved significant results with previous OT or other sensory interventions. Adrian's mother reported that he demonstrated atypical movement since he was three months old. He was constantly moving, rolling and rubbing his body against surfaces and caregivers. At six months, he started gagging and vomiting, which, not surprisingly, was followed by oral aversion and extreme picky eating.

When I met Adrian, he was moving constantly and had difficulty sitting and attending to quiet tasks. He was walking on his toes and banging his head. In order to fall asleep, Adrian needed to move and push his body against his parents. It took him one to two hours to fall asleep every night. He would wake up often during the night, especially when a parent's touch was removed.

One of the most difficult things for his parents was Adrian's extreme sensitivity and resistance during daily care activities. They were unable to bathe him or brush his teeth, and his curly hair was long and tangled like a lion's mane. He'd say that lotion was hurting him. Adrian was also sensitive to sounds. He cried, hid and covered his ears when the blender or the vacuum went on. He was extremely agitated and unhappy for large parts of his day and so were his sleep-deprived parents.

When his parents began QST, it was very difficult because Adrian kept running around the room and was unable to lie down. *An important part of his parents' QST training was learning how to meet his energy needs by using many repetitions of fast and light tapping in the movements down the back from head to feet (like Movements 5 and 6 in the sensory protocol). By doing so, they were able to gradually bring his energy down (out of his head and into his body) and help him calm his nervous energy and relax.* He was also very sensitive at the ears and his *mom learned how to alternate between fast tapping (clearing) and slow pressing (filling) movements until he was able to tolerate touch in that area.* After about five weeks, Adrian started to accept the entire QST routine, and it was much easier for Mom to do it on her own. He started to ask for "tap-tap" and frequently asked if Ms. Tap-Tap (me) was coming, greeting me with a big smile when I arrived. He positioned himself for the QST session and we completed the 12 movements with greater ease each time.

A week after starting daily QST, Adrian drank orange juice for the first time and willingly washed his hands! The next week, he agreed to take a bath and fell asleep within 20–30 minutes of QST. In the third week, Adrian started to feed himself and to cooperate with tooth brushing, and his speech became clearer as he was able to slow down. Grandma even started to help during the nightly QST routine as she noticed the quick and obvious positive changes in Adrian.

After five months of daily QST, Adrian's scores on the *Sense and Self-Regulation Checklist* all came down into the typical ranges. Adrian was asking for "tap-tap" every night. He was also asking to take a bath, getting haircuts on a regular basis and no longer resisting any grooming activities. He was trying and eating new foods (yes, broccoli!) and enjoyed cooking activities with his parents. He went to sleep on his own in his own bed and slept through the night. He was no longer constipated and got fully toilet trained. He stopped crashing and banging his head and was no longer bothered by sounds. He enjoyed a friend's birthday party for the first time (he used to scream on such occasions), accepted limits without meltdowns and followed directions much better. *When he became hyperactive on occasion, a quick clearing (tapping) down his arms and legs would bring him back to calm.* Calmer and less anxious throughout the day and across settings, Adrian became very engaged and talkative and participated in all activities at preschool, including sitting and completing table-top tasks.

Adrian's parents continued the daily QST for about two years, in which time he continued to do well. In the third year, he only received the QST routine at times of big transitions, such as for two weeks when starting kindergarten. Infrequently, when overly excited, Adrian may have a short episode of jumping and crashing, but other than that, his parents do not have any concerns. He adjusted well to his new kindergarten classroom (with no special supports), and he eats a large variety of foods, including veggies! His mother stated that QST was of great significance to Adrian's overall development and to their family. She is happy to have QST as a tool she can always use to connect and relax together with her son. She would like to tell other parents (like you) that:

It pays to try QST. Even if you don't believe . . . try it as a time to bond with your child and provide one-to-one attention and you will definitely see positive changes with some time. It was difficult at times, . . . but . . . as time went by it became more fun and time to bond with him.

Wishing you similar experiences in your own QST journey,
Orit Tal-Atzili, OTD, OTR/L
Certified QST Trainer and Master Trainer

Rockville, Maryland, USA

www.qsti.org/meet-our-master-trainers.html

To read more about Dr. Tal-Atzili's program see Appendix F – QST in Early Intervention.

Week 13

Getting Comfortable and Noticing More

The routine seems so natural to me now. It's how I touch my child anyway.

Kari M, mother of a 5-year-old

Dear parents,

Congratulations on passing the three-month mark! Now that you and your child are getting used to the routine of the daily treatment, we hope that you are able to relax into it more and more for yourself. This is one of the many wonderful and often unanticipated benefits of doing QST. Parents tell us that they may start the treatment feeling tired but are afterwards surprised to find they feel refreshed. That's actually what medical research has shown – that the person giving a massage gets similar benefits as the person who is receiving it. It's the same, and even more true, for QST.

QST has brought us closer. He is much more affectionate and cuddly now.

Mary J, mother of a 5-year-old

Many parents also tell us that as they find the calm to help their child, they also discover that their own senses open up and they start to notice new things during this process. An experience that parents sometimes notice during the first few months of QST is one of strange smells and tastes while doing the treatment. This is most probably a signal of your own increasing attunement. Your child's body is clearing his system of unwanted substances that he may have taken in from food or the environment. As his circulation improves, it is not unusual for your child to flush and cleanse his system during the first few months. Don't be unsettled, if the taste or smell becomes too strong, open a window and keep going.

When I did his QST last week, I could taste something in my mouth that seemed metallic.

Andrew C, father of a 4-year-old

As you come to relax, your child's body is not the only thing you'll begin to notice more acutely. You will become more open to experiencing your own body and the rhythms that you follow. At this point, parents sometimes wonder whether Qigong could be useful for themselves as well. In fact, Qigong is one of the five branches of Traditional Chinese Medicine, and people in China have used Qigong movements and exercises to improve health and vitality for thousands of years. These exercises really do work if you do them consistently every day. Research shows that they decrease stress, improve energy and strengthen the immune system. If you are interested, we have created a 15-minute Qigong exercise routine especially for our parents and therapists. You can take a look at the bookstore on our website: www.qsti.org/product/self-care-qigong-dvd-download/. If you take the time to do this every day, we promise you'll feel the rewards.

QST is a treatment that helps the helper. In fact, becoming more open to both your child's and your own internal cues and needs is one of the chief goals of the routine. We know that parents often feel that there is just not another minute in their day. But the more that you care for yourself, whether it's a personal Qigong practice, yoga, a trip to the gym or getting your own massage, the more energy you will have to care for your child! Give yourself permission to take care of yourself as a top priority!

All the best,

Louisa and Linda

Week 14

Widening the Circle of QST Helpers

Dear parents,

By this point, you and your child have settled into a comfortable routine, and he is probably able to tolerate a lot more touch. So, this would be a great time to share the QST technique with other members of the family, including your parenting partner, other adults in the household or even siblings. Adding the loving hands and intentions of other family members can bring even greater benefits! Most importantly, it gives one parent a necessary break on the days when their own health or energy is in need of rest.

There are many ways to include another adult to lend a supporting hand during QST. For example, you can alternate repetitions of each QST movement, or you may choose to work together (four hands) as you do a particular movement. The following list provides suggestions for effective ways to include a supportive and helping hand in each of the 12 QST movements. As you work together using these hands-on techniques, be sure to watch for your child's body and behavioral cues that show he is receptive to this new type of touch. If not, adapt your touch technique so you are always moving your child toward the relax-relate mode. (see Weeks 9, 10 and 28 for cues to look for.)

How to include helping hands in each QST movement:

Key: Never restrain

Support hands can be used to provide a sense of safety through warm, attuned containment. This is where your own sense of calm is important. If your child shows an escalating stress response, especially in the beginning weeks, you may need to take a brief cuddle break before resuming the movement.

---

1. **Making a connection.** This is a movement where both partners can work together, one parent on each side of the child, doing pressing movements in unison from the shoulder, down the arm to the hand and fingers. [See Appendix H for link to online video: *QST With Two Parents or Caregivers.*]

2. **Relax chest.** It can be very helpful to have a second helper place a supporting hand, resting it warmly on the lower belly. If your child's knees tend to come up, the second partner can use warm, calm resting hands on the thighs.

3. **Belly circles.** If your child has constipation, a second person can pat down the front of his legs while you do the belly circles (start with counterclockwise circles). If the problem is diarrhea, have the second person press slowly down the front of the child's legs instead of patting (start with clockwise circles). For any of the movements when working on the lower body, a support hand resting warmly on the belly can help. Even very young children in the family can participate in this way.

4. **Down the legs – front.** While you are doing this movement, it can be very helpful to have a second adult place one supporting hand resting warmly over the heart and the other hand resting warmly on the lower belly.

5. **Down the back – one hand** and . . .

6. **Down the back – two hands.** Here, one parent can pat down the head and back while the other adult/sibling picks up this movement at the hips and carries it down the lower body to the heels, creating one fluid movement from top to bottom. Working this way can be very helpful in bringing your child's energy down the body, especially if he is having a hard time laying on the table, his feet float up or his legs kick. If your child's legs kick or fly up, one parent can pat down from the top of the head to the toes, while the other applies slow-deep-rhythmic pressure down the back of the legs (but steps aside when the first parent brings the movement down to the heels).

7. **Down the sides.** If your child has a lot of discomfort around the ears or has had a lot of ear infections, having one person pat around the ear while the other pats on the top of the shoulder can be really helpful in clearing out the ears.

8. **Ear to hand.** Much the same approach can be followed here, except that instead of the second person patting only on the top of the shoulders, they continue the movement down the arms.

9. **Fingers.** It's often helpful for a second person to gently place their hand on the child's chest. The support hand should firmly but gently rest over the heart. Hold the intention of love and energy in your mind, picturing that love and energy moving from your heart through your hand to your child's heart. In fact, for any of the movements when working on the upper body, if your child is receptive to this type of touch, a support hand resting warmly on the chest can be very quieting and bring a sense of calm.

10. **Relax legs** and

11. **Toes.** While you are doing both of these movements, it can be very helpful to have a second adult rest a supporting hand warmly on the lower belly. This will help your child make a connection between his belly and lower legs and help to advance his gross motor skills.

12. **Nourish and Integrate – Rhythmic Wave.** Supporting hands on your child's chest and belly during this movement can really help his body to stabilize and integrate the entire QST

routine. Sometimes when this happens, a child will take a parent's hand and lay it on his forehead, face, chest or belly. Trust what your child is telling you with this action. He will often show you just how to best use your supporting hands. By the way, the usefulness of the extra hands on the chest and belly is not limited to Movement 12. Feel free to apply this very helpful technique whenever your child needs extra support!

Many hands not only make light work but also boost the effectiveness of the routine and bring the family closer together. Enjoy!

All our best,

Louisa and Linda

QST for Daily Regulation – Weeks 15–20

Week 15

QST to Support Emotional Regulation

Reflections From a QST Master Trainer

Dear parents,

Children with sensory and behavioral challenges, particularly those who are over-sensitive or over-reactive to sensory stimulation, often really struggle with self-regulation, self-control and managing the big feelings that affect their behaviors. More and more, we are beginning to understand how important learning to self-regulate is in order for a child to master self-control. It lays the foundations for a range of future skills throughout life. This includes emotional well-being, developing good relationships, academic learning and being able to control emotions.

In my experience as an OT and QST Therapist, persevering with the QST routine every day with your child assists in the important development of these fundamental skills (i.e., self -regulation, attention and concentration for learning and improved self-control). Self-regulation is your ability to understand and manage your energy levels, behavior, feelings and reactions to the things happening in your environment. It helps your child to:

- ignore distractions so that they can focus and pay attention to listen and learn.
- be able to make friends and develop social skills to get along well with others.
- control their impulses and behave in socially acceptable ways.
- Learn how to cope with big feelings and express their emotions in appropriate ways
- Be able to self-soothe and calm after getting excited, frustrated, angry or upset
- Make good choices about their behavior and learn how to behave in different situations

A child's ability to regulate their emotions, reactions and behavior is critical to their ability to develop and use self-regulation skills. This then forms the foundation for the development of self-control. If a child is feeling overwhelmed by all the sensory stimulation they are exposed to during the day, or if they are under-sensitive and struggling to register what is going on in their environment, QST makes a significant impact on their ability to participate, deal with strong emotions or get along with others around them. When children are easily frustrated, upset or angry, it can also make it difficult to listen, remember rules and stay focused on learning.

DOI: 10.4324/9781003360421-19

We also know that sleep is very important for learning, and a lack of good sleep tends to exacerbate difficulties with self-regulation. QST helps to calm and restore balance to the nervous system. It gradually helps to alleviate sensory issues and improves the length and quality of your child's sleep. When you are doing Movement 2 on the chest and Movement 12 at the end of the routine, you are helping your child's nervous system to relax and learn what it feels like to be calm, quiet and focused. This in turn gradually helps them in times of stress to be able to self-soothe and calm themselves.

Children gradually start to develop more flexibility and the ability to stay calm and be less reactive in the face of situations that previously would have upset or emotionally overwhelmed them. This then makes it easier for them to engage in learning and interact and play with other children. As children's sensory issues decrease, their ability to respond more appropriately to sensory stimulation (visual, touch, sound, movement, taste and smell) improves. Self-regulation starts to become easier for them and children naturally begin to make more effective choices about how they behave. You will find that your child's ability to attend and concentrate also improves, along with their ability to manage and control their emotional reactions to big feelings.

Best wishes,

Sue Clayton, OT

QST Master Trainer, Australia

www.qsti.org/master-trainers/

Week 16

Sleep Problems

Chinese Medicine and Energy Flow

Dear parents,

Proper sleep is among the most important components of a child's daily cycle of regulation. QST understands problems with sleep and, in fact, all of the other self-regulatory milestones through the lens of Chinese medicine and energy flow or qi. You already have a common-sense appreciation of energy. You know when you have plenty of energy and when your energy is low. What might be new to you is how Chinese medicine describes the natural flow of energy throughout the body that has a direct impact on health and well-being.

From this perspective, when we sleep, the natural movement of energy is always downward (from head to toe) and inward (from the surface deeper into body). If energy is blocked and cannot flow downward into the body, it will remain trapped or blocked in the head. In the West, we intuit this in the terms we use: we calm 'down', settle 'down' and 'turn in' for the night. And when that energy is blocked in the head, we say: "I was 'up' all night" and "I couldn't settle down'". Children, by their very nature, have much more energy in their head area, and when all goes well, that energy moves freely throughout the body. But blocks in the flow can cause discomfort, "disease", dysregulation and a range of symptoms, including sleep problems. There are many things that can cause blocks to this healthy flow, including injury, stress, infections, irregular sleep, poor diet, toxins and harmful substances in the body.

In order for your child to fall asleep, the energy must be able to flow down from the head, through the neck and shoulders all the way down to the toes. But for kids with sensory problems, it is very common to find energy blocks related to sleep, at the base of the skull. The neck and shoulders are another common area where tight and knotted muscles can keep energy trapped in the head. Both the 'down the back' and 'extra neck clearing' movements are especially helpful to open the flow of energy and ease muscle tension in these areas. (See Chapter 8 – Movements 5, 6 and Optional Extra Neck Clearing Before Movement 5.) You will know that the energy is flowing downward and that sleep will improve when your child is able to naturally lay both her head and body down completely.

A different problem occurs if your child can fall asleep at night but wakes up three hours later. This means that although you have gotten the skin and surface muscles to soften and relax so your child can *fall* asleep, the even deeper layers of muscle are still blocked. The solution is simple: pay more attention to the deeper muscles of the neck and shoulders by first tapping into the nape of the neck with the pads of your fingertips (be careful of fingernails) until you feel the muscles soften and relax. (See the optional extra neck clearing technique just before Movement 5). Then, when doing 'down the sides' (Movement 7), pat for a longer time on the tops of the shoulders until they feel completely loose and bouncy under your hands. You may have to do this several days in a row, but once you are able to relax these deeper parts of her neck muscles, the block will clear and she should sleep through the night.

In the next weeks, we'll look at some other self-regulatory problems – listening, paying attention and tantrums – through this lens of energy flow and will show you how to address them with your daily QST.

Wishing you many good nights' sleep!

Louisa and Linda

Week 17

Listening Problems

Opening the Ears

Dear parents,

Problems with hearing and the ability to listen have a direct impact on your child's capacity to self-regulate and pay attention, so today, we take a look at the ears and the ability to listen from the perspective of blocked energy. Those blocks in and around the ears can create barriers to feeling and using the ears to listen, pay attention, learn and engage socially. You may have never thought about the skin and the muscles around the ears as having anything to do with hearing, but they actually do. Sensitivity to touch on and around the ears is one of the most common problems for children with immature sensory systems and can result in problems with listening. If you remember from Chapter 1, when we are in fight-flight-or-freeze mode, the muscles of the inner ear actually constrict and ears are tuned only to hear sounds related to threat; they are *not* tuned to hear sounds in the range of the spoken voice.

In our conversation about sleep problems last week, we saw how children with nervous systems that are easily tipped into survival mode tend to have problems where energy gets 'stuck' in the head and does not flow easily down into the rest of the body as it normally would. In the same way this can show up as sleep problems, it can also be seen in ear, hearing and listening problems, tense neck muscles and distracted attention.

How to help with QST. The patting and/or pressing motion that you use in the 'down the sides' and 'ear to hand' movements will help your child to feel more comfortable and receptive to touch around the ears. This can take a few weeks or months. The more sensitive your child is to touch, the longer it can take to normalize that touch. Patting will help to clear blocks, but if your child does not tolerate the patting motion, move to slower, deeper pressuring movements. Once she can tolerate the deeper pressing, then go back and try the patting motion again. Do not avoid the ears. It is your 'attuned' touch technique that over time will help to normalize the skin around the ears to touch.

But for the ears themselves, we need to go a bit deeper and do a bit more. We need to be sure that the muscles that attach on the side of the neck, just under and behind the ears, are completely soft and comfortable too. You can get to those muscles by tapping into them with the pads of your fingers and patting on the top of the shoulder at the same time. This is most easily done in the optional 'extra ear tapping' and the 'ear to hand' movements (see Chapter 8 – Movement 8). Tap under the ear with one hand and on the top of the shoulder with your other hand. It will speed up progress when you pat both simultaneously. This causes the whole muscle to vibrate and the block to shake loose. If two of you are giving the routine together, it can be very effective if one person taps under the ear while the other pats on top of the shoulder. You can see a demonstration of this in the online video instruction [see link in Appendix H] for Movement 8. (See also Weekly Letter 14 – Widening the Circle for QST Helpers, page 144.)

As you open energy flow in the skin and the deeper muscles of the neck, this also allows energy and circulation to flow more freely down the arms and into the fingers. So, as your child's hearing and listening improve, fingers that were previously sensitive to touch now also start to feel better. Wearing gloves and cutting nails become easier, and fine motor control can begin to improve. Next week, we will see how opening energy flow can also help resolve tantrums.

Our very best wishes,

Louisa and Linda

Week 18

Tantrums

Opening the Chest for Deep Relaxation

Dear parents,

This week, we focus on tantrums and on how opening the pathways for energy and circulation in the chest helps to reduce and resolve tantrums by regulating the sensory overload that caused them. In the last two weeks, we talked about opening energy pathways on the *outside* of the body (the back, ears and fingers), focusing on circulation closer to the surface. Today, we look at how the 'relax chest' movement helps to open energy pathways and circulation to the deeper organs and tissues *inside* the body, in the chest and belly. This QST movement engages both a deep relaxation response that calms the feelings of frustration and anxiousness that generate those tantrums while, over time, strengthening the inner capacities for self-soothing and self-regulation.

When we are stressed and shut down, the chest gets tight. When we are relaxed and open, the chest relaxes. Inside the chest, around the heart, is a huge network of tiny nerves that respond to deep exhales by relaxing and opening the chest so we can breathe more deeply. In the 'relax chest' movement, we stimulate that network of nerves to allow a deep relaxation response. When you place the warmth of your hands on your child's chest and use a rhythmic in-and-out pressure at the rate of a resting heartbeat, about 60 beats per minute, you mirror the relaxing sound of a mother's resting heartbeat in the womb. Think of these 60 pressures as delivering the love contained in 60 big hugs!

As you start rhythmically pressing in and out, your child's ribs may at first feel tight. That's okay. Focus on those tight areas, slow down and press gently in and out until you feel them begin to move and expand as the small muscles between the ribs relax. Our ribs are made to be flexible. When you take a really deep breath, they should expand and contract easily. Think about how much a child's ribs move when they take a really deep breath. Then try to use pressure deep enough to comfortably move the ribs just that much when you do the 'relax chest' movement. You want to feel the spaces between the ribs gently expanding and contracting.

Once the ribs relax under your hands, continue the movement down the chest until you've reached the bottom of the ribs (do not use pressure on the last floating rib). Watch your child's face. After a few minutes, you may see her yawn or reach up to rub her eyes. These are signs that the relaxation response has begun to turn on! After you've triggered this relaxation response several times, she will be able to trigger it for herself when she needs it, either to calm down or to get herself through a transition without having a meltdown. That's the goal!

My daughter is very sensitive and easily over-stimulated. The routine has really helped her be able to soothe herself. And the tantrums are basically gone!

Mom of a 3-year-old

Get to know where the tight areas are, and don't be afraid to continue pressing movements on those areas longer. Over time and with your help, her chest will be able to move in and out more freely. Occasionally, your child's hands may come up and touch your arm or cover your own hands. When this happens, stay even longer on that spot until her hands move away. This means you have opened up the circulation to her chest and she wants you to fill it up with your good energy.

Tantrums and outbursts reflect a child's inability to contain and express deep and often confusing feelings. Once circulation and energy have opened in the chest, children can access and contain those emotions with less fear of overwhelm, which means that as the energy is restored, the need for tantrums is reduced. But opening up the chest may also lead to the release of some other unexpected but deep emotions. The chest is a place where a child can hold grief, shame and other deep feelings, and the 'relax chest' movement is focused on opening these areas so the feelings can be released. When she relaxes, she may become aware of the feelings that were held there. So, it's quite natural that at some point, you may see your child release a few tears or other emotions. Don't be afraid of the tears! Allowing and even encouraging these feelings to come out will help them to pass. We'll tell you more about how to work with that in Weekly Letter 40 – Release of Emotions During QST and Weekly Letter 41 – Emotional Bubble – How to Help.

Good work!

Louisa and Linda

Week 19

Regulating Digestion and Elimination

Opening and Strengthening Flow to the Belly

Dear parents,

Regulating good digestion and elimination depends on a proper flow of energy and circulation to the belly. A huge network of nerves in the belly – over one hundred million nerve cells – helps to regulate digestion and orchestrate turning your child's food into energy and nutrients for growth. Physical signs that the belly isn't working properly can be obvious: poor appetite, reflux, diarrhea and constipation. QST can go a long way to help, first with recommendations for what you put *inside* your child's body (nutritious food) and then with the touch techniques that help you to channel energy flow to the belly through the daily routine. You already know how to move that energy by the way you adjust the belly movements for diarrhea or constipation. (To strengthen your child's belly and fill up her energy reserves, look back to Weekly Letter 14 – Widening the Circle of QST Helpers.) And you may have even seen the dark green bowel movements that tell you that the body has expelled old waste and begun to improve digestion. So, let's now focus first on the good food you provide.

Good nutrition is important for all children, and that includes eating healthy, home-prepared food. But for a child who has problems with learning and behavior, it becomes doubly important. Processed and packaged foods contain man-made chemicals that your child's body cannot turn into brain food, and these chemicals can hang around, causing problems with learning and behavior. If your child has reflux, it is especially important that you avoid ice and be sure to serve food that is warm and cooked. Basically, the stomach is a muscle that mashes the food so that it can be further digested. But ice water cools down the stomach, turning it into a stiff, frozen muscle that doesn't work well. Instead of going down, food goes back up, leading to reflux and vomiting. For children with compromised digestion, serving cold or raw food creates extra work for the stomach because it takes more energy to warm cold food and drinks and to process raw vegetables. Just think about how long it takes to cook them! So, if your child's digestive system is weak, don't feed her iced, cold or raw food until her system gets stronger. Take that load off her digestion by providing warm and cooked food and no ice! Yes, they can have fruit, but only after the meal or as a snack – not as the main meal.

Then, once you get the organs of digestion working smoothly with diet and the QST movements, you can focus on something even deeper – strong emotions. The belly, from the perspective of Chinese medicine, is where we hold the emotions of fear and anger. As you are working in this area, your child may release momentary 'bubbles' that express these emotions. Just stay calm, reassure your child by lovingly and confidently saying, "You're okay, you're okay" and confidently keep working on the area. This tells your child it's okay to feel those emotions and it will help to release them. Your child will be better off for having felt them and then let them go. Unless circumstances are unusual, these bubbles won't happen more than once or twice.

Once your child's belly is relaxed and digestion is working well, you will see that she is getting the energy she needs from her food. Good digestion and elimination resume, and before long, you will notice how much your child grows physically.

Best wishes,

Louisa and Linda

Week 20

Reading Body and Behavioral Cues – Perspectives From Chinese Medicine

Reflections From a QST Master Trainer

Dear parent,

Welcome to the soothing medicine that is QST. My observations of children who receive the QST routine from their parent confirm that the young body is quite responsive to healing touch. As this book conveys, helping your child become comfortable with the daily routine is facilitated by simple techniques such as patting and pressing or changing the pressure or speed of the movements in response to cues your child provides such as squirming or giggling.

Once the QST routine is well-established in your family's routine and your child has indicated that they are comfortable with your technique, then other bodily responses beyond squirming and wiggling may arise. Often, these responses are a good indication that you are making solid progress. I will describe now some other responses that I've seen and, since I am an acupuncturist, I will explain how Chinese medicine understands these responses in the process of healing.

Chinese medicine is rich in metaphor. We understand that the healthy body experiences a free flow of energy. Children host deep reservoirs of this vital energy, and in the healthy child, that energy moves freely. Sometimes when providing QST, parents will notice that their child's body is moving in a way that is responsive to their touch. For example, some children, while laying facedown, will kick their legs or lift their back – this is a response to the experience of energy moving in their bodies. The kick helps shift the energy down the legs and grounds the child. Others will twist – either right to left or left to right – we see this in Chinese medicine as a way of harmonizing the energy. These are natural moves the child makes in response to the QST movements. Others will stretch – if you have ever had a stretching routine, you may have had the experience of your body moving in ways that help you to regulate yourself. Your child will do the same. Consider these actions as a form of collaboration – your child's body has its own intelligence about how to cooperate with your touch treatment.

Once your regular routine is established, you will find that your child participates fully. By naming and identifying these kinds of actions as your child's offering helpful contributions to the routine, you empower your child to work with you in harmony. QST becomes a playful collaboration. You build respect for the wisdom inherent in your child's physical form.

Maria Broderick, EdD, MOAM, LicAc

Director of Clinical Education, Associate Professor

New England School of Acupuncture

QST Master Trainer

www.qsti.org/master-trainers/

Staying Consistent – Weeks 21–25

Week 21

Making it Through the 'Dog Days'

Dear parents,

At this point, you may find yourself in the 'dog days' with your QST and feel tempted to cut back on the consistency of the daily routine. Not every parent will experience this, but some will, so we think it's important to help you meet the challenges should they arise. Since dog days can look and feel different for different families depending on their experience, we thought we'd describe two common ways this feeling might show up and give you suggestions to keep moving through it. Typically, parents grow tired and frustrated when they've either seen very exciting success early but now find that progress has started to slow or if they've experienced precious little in the way of change after putting in a lot of effort. But whether you've experienced early successes or not, any slowdown can be frustrating and even demoralizing.

Let's begin with the parent who saw early positive results. Because early success can feel exciting and motivating, a slowdown can feel like you've gotten all you can from the routine. Some parents naturally let the daily routine slip at this point, but when your child begins to regress, you are quickly reminded of the importance of consistency. This is the time to remember that staying consistent to integrate and solidify those early successes is just as important as achieving the new ones. And harder still is trusting that the consistency will bring new successes. At these times, it helps to remember the progress you have made, and you may now be taking progress for granted: "Oh, yeah, he used to not go to sleep until 2:00 am, now he's falling asleep at 9:00 pm." Or you may realize, "Wow, he hasn't had a meltdown in weeks." Reviewing your small successes will remind you how far you've come, re-energize your commitment and help get you through.

Other parents may feel that by this time, they've not seen much improvement at all and may doubt that the treatment will work for their child. Maybe your child couldn't lie down for the treatment, and you've had to chase him around and give it in stages throughout the day. Maybe the meltdowns are still happening on a regular basis. This is another way dog days can look – exhausted, confused and frustrated. If this is you, take heart – if you are doing the treatment correctly, doing it every day, tuning in to your child's responses and changing from patting to pressing as needed, you *will* get results. Children are all different and some will make smaller improvements more slowly. But all will progress. It helps to remember the small changes.

DOI: 10.4324/9781003360421-20

But whether you've had early success or not, parents can at times get completely overwhelmed. If you are not sure you are doing this right, if you are confused about your child's responses and how to adapt the technique or if you're simply not seeing much progress, you may need some extra help. You can get coaching and support from a certified QST trainer through the Qigong Sensory Training Institute at www.QSTI.org/finding-a-qst-trainer/. For families without access to a local QST trainer, online coaching is available. So reach out, get help and don't give up!

The main point is, if you are experiencing the dog days, shake things up a little. Recommit to doing the treatment every day, get another family member to do it with you or alternate days, make a list of all of the small improvements to keep yourself motivated and get help and support if you need it. This is exactly the point to renew your commitment. Our research studies have consistently shown that parents who maintain the daily routine see the strongest results. We know you can keep going. We know you will see positive results if you do. After all, you've come a long way already!

All our best,

Louisa and Linda

Week 22

The Four Risk Periods for Dropping the Daily QST Routine

Dear parents,

Many years of experience has taught us that there are four major risk periods when parents are most likely to give up and discontinue the treatment. We feel it is important that you know the signs of these risk periods so you don't mis-read the cues and give up too soon. These periods can pop up at the outset if you aren't adapting your technique to your child's touch sensitivities. They may also occur when you have correctly adapted to those needs but the needs have now changed and you missed that signal. Or the risk of giving up can creep in when progress slows to a crawl and you decide prematurely that there are no more gains to be made. We want to forewarn you about each of these periods so you don't give up before your child has achieved all the benefits possible from your diligent work.

The four risk periods:

1. **When you first begin.** If your child shows a lot of resistance when you first start the program, it's easy to think that he doesn't like QST or, more commonly, that it just doesn't work for him. Both conclusions are mistaken. If your child is struggling and not accepting the routine at the beginning, it is most likely that you have not yet found the right technique, meaning the right speed, rhythm or weight of your hand that will make it possible for him to be receptive to the movements without triggering a struggle. You will need to modify your technique to make it tolerable for your child. Here is what to do!

- Re-read the instructions for the particular movement(s) that cause your child to struggle or resist (Chapter 8 – QST Sensory Protocol – Step-by-Step Instructions).
- Review the online video instructions for those specific movements [link in Appendix H, page 221].
- See Weekly Letters to parents for suggestions on how to work through resistances (Part III: Weekly Letters 3, 4 and 11).

- Also, see *QST 12-Movement Troubleshooting Guide* (Appendix B) and "How to Work Through the Difficult Spots" (Chapter 10).
- Don't give up! Again and again, we have seen parents work through what initially seemed like insurmountable struggles and find success and improvements for their child.

2. **After a few months.** If you have a child with an under-sensitive sensory system (i.e., unresponsive to touch or doesn't feel pain when injured) you may experience a sudden period of challenging behaviors as touch starts to feel more normal to him. It is common for an under-sensitive child to switch to over-sensitive as they start to feel new and more sensation in their skin. In fact, this is a huge sign of progress! If this happens, you may miss this as the positive sign that it is. In fact, it's normal to think that QST has stopped working or to even feel it has made things worse. Both conclusions are wrong. One big tip-off that your child has entered this next stage is that he begins to cry when he is injured when he has never done that before. These shifts from under- to over-sensitive are typical and show positive progress on the road to your ultimate goal – normalized touch sensitivity. The over-sensitive stage can last for a few weeks, so it is best to be prepared. To help your child get through this stage faster and more easily, modify your touch technique as soon as you notice this shift. Read more about this transition in Weekly Letters 4, 6, 7, 8, and 12.

3. **After a major developmental shift.** Not all new challenging behavior is cause for despair. For example, you might conclude that the routine has stopped working because your child, for no apparent reason, starts testing you, saying "no" a lot. But that could also be a good sign! When QST improves your child's sensory system to a certain point, he will begin to develop a more independent sense of self. That's because the skin and the improved sense of touch are giving him information about all parts of his body, helping him to experience a more integrated whole-body sense. Now he can feel his will – a will that he wants to test against yours! This is a very normal developmental stage and a wonderful achievement on your part! At this point, you just need to switch your parenting style to help him understand that he has choices, but he doesn't control the world! See more tips about parenting this stage in Weekly Letter 20 – Staying the Course, Weekly Letter 43 – Stuck in Stress Mode and Weekly Letter 44 – The Need for Predictability.

4. **When progress levels off.** There are times when a child's progress is no longer as dramatic as it had been in the beginning. At those times, your daily QST may begin to fall off your priority list because you've decided that your child has gotten all of the benefits that were possible. You can probably guess by now that this too is often the wrong conclusion! First of all, normal growth and development don't follow a continuous steady upward trend. These processes move in spurts and plateaus, so a 'stop' is often only the next 'spurt' getting ready to begin. Secondly, growth happens very slowly and is easy to miss on a daily basis. Then, for example, when a relative who visits only occasionally points the changes out to you, you can see them for the first time. Our research shows that parents who continued the daily routine and were able to adapt through several plateaus or slow periods discovered that their children continued to make steady progress in development through the two-year period of the study.

We hope these resources and supports will help you to not give up or give in to the feelings of frustration and discouragement, and trust that good things are often happening even when you can't see them right away.

Best wishes,
Louisa and Linda

Week 23

Staying the Course

Reflections from a QST Master Trainer

Dear parents,

Sometimes when starting QST with your child, there is a 'honeymoon phase', especially for children with sensory processing difficulties. At first, they may respond really well and cooperate when you indicate it is time for QST. Hopefully, this continues on a daily basis and your Qigong time is nothing but positive and bond-building between you and your beloved son or daughter. However, life often gets in the way, your child may start avoiding the treatment for no apparent reason and it can suddenly become difficult to remain consistent in carrying out the daily routine.

Many children with sensory issues try to find ways to control their routines at home, especially if they are using much of their energy to hold it together at school. After the newness has worn off, your child may avoid, resist, ask for just parts of the QST movements, or demonstrate other behaviors to deter the routine that you have established. If and when this happens, don't give up! Let your child feel like he or he has a part in controlling the situation by giving choices:

"Would you like to do Qigong in your room or in the living room?"
"Do you want to brush your teeth before or after your QST?"

Another method to ingrain QST into your child's routine is to choose a special blanket that is used only for Qigong and/or to have calming music playing softly. You can also make a fun game by cutting up a copy of the *QST Sensory Movement Chart* into squares and let your child hand you the one that comes next. After a while, they can verbally tell you what is next (maybe you can pretend to forget).

Undoubtedly, many obstacles will arise that can sway parents from completing the daily QST routine. Life happens! Try your best, forgive yourself and get back on track. You have the power in your healing hands to help your child succeed in his or her everyday life. Increasing self-regulation will flow over into better focus in school, improved relationships with peers and adults, better sleep and digestion and independence with everyday tasks.

I am cheering for you!
Best wishes,
Adrienne
Adrienne Harvey, MS, OTR/L
QST Master Trainer
Wyoming, USA
www.QSTI.org/master-trainers/

Week 24

A Skeptical Parent Comes to Believe

A Mother's Story

Dear parents,

I first heard about QST from my son's OT a few months after he started school. He had just turned six. Initially I was skeptical; it sounded like one of those mystic energy healing things I definitely didn't believe in. Then the OT showed me some of the scientific studies that found QST was effective, and I was intrigued. By the time of our next OT meeting a week later, I had bought a copy of the book and read it and had copies of all of the studies that had been published. I was starting to be convinced. The scientific studies made all of the difference to me.

At that time, my son was having a very difficult time adjusting to school. He was hitting the staff and I was worried he would be thrown out of school, but my house was very clean because I was so anxious I couldn't sleep and was up most nights cleaning! He had many sensory challenges – hyper-sensitivity to light, sound and some touch (he wouldn't wear socks). He also didn't like it when other children cried, including babies. At the park, we had to rush to be near him if a child cried as there was a risk of him hitting the child in an effort to stop the crying. A few times we were not fast enough, and he did hit children at the beach, park and school. He was not sleeping well, would sometimes take a long time to fall asleep or he would wake up in the middle of the night and not be able to go back to sleep. I always heard him, so I didn't sleep much either. He would have some spectacular tantrums that could last for what seemed like forever. I used to call him my Ferrari because he could go from 0–60 in a few seconds. Food was another challenge; he was a very fussy eater.

When I started using QST, to be honest I wasn't expecting much. I decided I would commit to doing the daily routine faithfully for the five months indicated in the studies I'd read, and I was going to evaluate it then. Around Christmas, my son's class went to the nearby shopping mall to visit Santa. One day, his teacher was telling me about the trip and commenting that he loved fries. She had given him fries from McDonald's at the mall. My first reaction was horror at the fact that she had introduced my son to the very symbol of junk food! Then I thought, "Wait a minute, he ate them?" My son, who only ate a handful of things with a particular texture. Until he was three years old, I had to puree his food. I think it was then that I allowed myself a faint glimmer of hope that this treatment might actually help him. Those fries represented a major step in a long journey for us.

At the end of the five months, he was wearing socks, tantrums were less frequent both at home and at school, he was sleeping much better and had even started playing around with words to make simple jokes! Two years later, we still do QST several times a week. It seems to help him. I would tell new parents that QST works! It has been tested in many studies. There's not much you can do wrong with it. All you have to do is spend a few minutes every day with your child and that time together is very special.

Many thanks,
Sarah (mother)

Week 25

Still Hyper? Diet is Key

Dear parents,

There are many other factors outside of QST that can impact sensory and behavioral growth. At the top of that list is diet. In today's world, our foods contain more and more additives. Packaged foods for children are highly processed, loaded with sugar and contain artificial food colorings, flavorings and other toxic chemicals. While these additives are not good for any child, they pose an even greater problem for children with sensory issues, who are often slower to process these chemicals. The impact of these toxins is stronger and lasts longer in their bodies. It's easy to overlook the importance of diet. Eliminating these additives can clear away invisible roadblocks to your child's health and speed up improvements in a dramatic way.

Multiple studies in recent years have shown how children are adversely affected by food additives. At least one recent study has shown that artificial food coloring and flavors cause hyperactivity, even in some children without attentional or behavioral problems. And a larger study conducted in England with several thousand children reported that red dye in food caused hyperactive behavior.

The story of a child in one of our own studies perfectly illustrates how these additives can affect behavior. This little girl, with high-functioning autism and lots of sensory issues, talked non-stop and had almost no awareness of how her behavior affected other children. Her teacher complained that her non-stop talking disrupted classroom activities and that other children didn't want to be her friend. This little girl ate an almost constant diet of soda, chips, candy and fast foods.

Her mom decided to remove all of the junk food from her diet. She switched the entire family over to whole foods (no more chips, no more candy) and offered them water instead of soda. She made simple, homemade, nutritious meals and offered fruit for snacks. The change in her daughter was like night and day. She calmed down, started listening and no longer talked non-stop. Her school very soon reported the same positive changes. While this is a pretty extreme example, it does illustrate how eliminating highly processed, sugar laden foods containing artificial colors and flavorings and moving to a simple and nutritious whole-food diet can be a crucially important part of your child's health. So, if your child continues to exhibit hyperactive behaviors, even after these many weeks of QST, take a closer look at your child's diet and take out the sugar, food coloring and processed food for a few weeks. We think you will be very pleased with the results and that you may also see faster progress with your QST.

Very best wishes,

Louisa and Linda

Noticing Changes – Marking Progress – Weeks 26–32

Week 26

Noticing Changes and Progress Over Time

Dear parents,

One striking thing that we have noticed over the years is that it's not always easy for parents to see the real changes occurring in their children on a day-to-day basis. There are a couple of reasons why this is not unusual. First, while some changes may be obvious, like improvements in sleep, most improvements come slowly, little-by-little or day-by-day, so they are easy to overlook. Second, what you experience today feels like the new normal and it's easy to forget where you started. We quite naturally focus on the problems and challenges in front of us today and forget how much worse those problems felt weeks or months ago.

It is also natural to not connect changes that you see today with what you've been doing to make that change happen. It's similar to when we exercise or lose weight. We don't always notice the day-to-day changes, but when we meet a friend we haven't seen in a while, they tell us the changes they see and immediately bring the picture of our own success into sharper focus. That tendency to not notice growth is why it is so important to pause from time to time to look carefully at where you are and how you've succeeded. Recognizing the changes builds your confidence in what you are doing and encourages you to engage more fully and comfortably in the movements. And that change in you is something your child, who is so tuned in to your feelings and intentions, will also notice and feel *with* you. Next week, we will have you fill out a second set of checklists and the progress chart for a mid-year check. Once you've completed these, we'll show you how to compare your 'start date' scores with your 'mid-year-check' scores to see how far you have come and identify the areas to focus on in the months to come.

Best wishes,

Louisa and Linda

DOI: 10.4324/9781003360421-21

Week 27

Mid-Year Check-In

Dear parents,

When you began QST six months ago, we had you complete two checklists – the *Sense and Self-Regulation Checklist* and the *Parenting Stress Index* – as well as the *QST Progress Chart*. At this point, halfway into your one-year journey with QST, it can be easy to forget what your child's behavioral and sensory picture was when you started. That is why we had you complete the set of 'start date' checklists, to give you a baseline picture of your child's strengths, difficulties and challenges. But don't look back at those scores until you complete your mid-year check; then, you can look back to compare.

You may remember that the *Sense and Self-Regulation Checklist* measures the degree of your child's touch and regulation difficulties. The *Parenting Stress Index* evaluates the level of your own stress and worry about those problems. And the *QST Progress Chart* gives you the do-it-yourself chart with a 'picture' of the major regulation milestones and sensory areas. Now, without looking back at your beginning checklists, we are asking you to complete these same measures again so you can compare how the scores have changed over the last six months. You already know that your child has improved. These scores will show you exactly how much. This is what scientists do to prove that something does – or does not – work. It is also how our QST therapists track a child's progress. As a parent, you can use the same approach. Let's take a look at how to compare your start date and mid-year check to see how far you have come.

Instructions to complete mid-year checklists

Please go now to complete the two mid-year checklists at the end of this letter. (You can also download and print out a copy of the forms – See link in Appendix H, page 221 – as many parents have found them a useful tool to share with their child's medical, school or intervention team.) When you have those scores, come back to this page to record them and compare with your start date scores.

Now, let's compare today's scores with those from the beginning. Please look back to the end of Chapter 7 (page 60–62) to find your beginning scores and fill in the blanks below:

Sense and Self-Regulation Checklist

> **Start Date** Total Score: _____
> **Mid-Year Check** Total Score: _____

Parent Stress Index

> **Start Date** Total Score: _____
> **Mid-Year Check** Total Score: _____

What did you find? Did the scores go down? Depending on how severe your child's sensory, self-regulation and behavioral difficulties were to begin with, the current scores may have come down a lot or a little. Now, let's take a look at what each of those scores mean.

For scores that came down on the *Sense and Self-Regulation Checklist*: A lower score means that your child's problems with touch and self-regulation have improved. The areas of her body that were over-sensitive to touch are calming down, while those areas that were under-sensitive – that is, they had very little feeling – are now awakening so she can feel them. Touch is becoming more normalized. Your skilled touch has opened up her awareness of her body and she can experience her surroundings in more regulated ways.

For scores that came down on the *Parent Stress Index*: A lower score here means that parenting has become less stressful than it was before starting QST. But you probably don't need those scores to tell you that! While that lower score is generally a good thing, sometimes a higher score can actually be a positive sign too. How? We found that it indicates a temporary increase in what we might call 'positive stress' as parents become more aware of what to look for. This 'helpful' stress arises from a focusing of skills and intention, leading to greater parent efficacy and improved scores.

I didn't even know I should be worried about these things – it's just the way things were. Now I'm stressing about potty training because we're actually working on potty training! Before I didn't even know it was possible so why stress about it?

Mother of a 4-year-old

Instructions to complete the Mid-Year Progress Chart

Just as you did at the beginning, fill in the *QST Progress Chart* below, circling the number that best reflects your child's current capacities for regulation in each column. Connect the scores with a line, and don't forget to include the same items you may have previously written in on the two extra lines on the far-right side.

QST Progress Chart - Mid-Year Check

Sleep	Digestion Elimination	Focus Attention	Self Regulation	Social Connection	Tantrums Aggression	Touch Sensitivity	/	/
10	10	10	10	10	10	10	10	10
9	9	9	9	9	9	9	9	9
8	8	8	8	8	8	8	8	8
7	7	7	7	7	7	7	7	7
6	6	6	6	6	6	6	6	6
5	5	5	5	5	5	5	5	5
4	4	4	4	4	4	4	4	4
3	3	3	3	3	3	3	3	3
2	2	2	2	2	2	2	2	2
1	1	1	1	1	1	1	1	1

Self-Regulation Milestones

Figure 17.1 **QST Progress Chart Mid-Year Check** – circle the number in each column that reflects your child's current capabilities. "10" is very positive/no difficulty, and "1" is most difficult. Then connect the circles to complete the sensory and self-regulation "picture".

Now, look back to the start date *QST Progress Chart* you completed in Chapter 7 (page 58) that reflected your child's capacities for regulation before beginning QST. Using a different color pen or pencil, duplicate those numbers and the connecting line onto this present chart.

How to Read Your Mid-Year Scores

Comparing your beginning and 'mid-year' scores gives you a bird's eye view of the progress your child has made to date. It gives you a visual picture of the degree of improvement there has been in each of the areas of regulation. Comparing your scores over time may also help to focus your attention on areas of progress that you may have overlooked or those that need more attention. To better understand how to read your child's chart, let's take a look at an example of a chart that was completed by a parent, one that includes both *Start Date* and *Mid-Year Check* scores combined.

Example of a parent completed Mid-Year Check

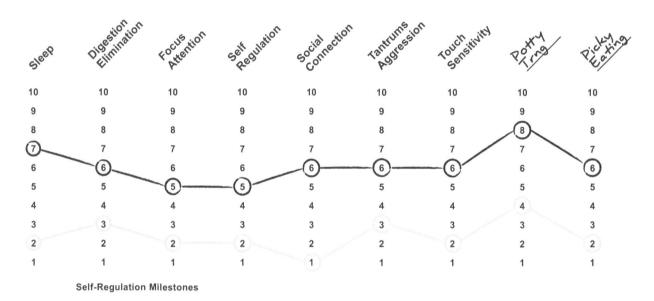

Figure 17.2 **Example of a Mid-Year Check - QST Progress Chart** completed by a parent with Start Date scores (circled numbers with lighter line at bottom of chart) and Mid-Year Check scores (darker line above).

The Start Date scores, circled and connected with the lighter line at the bottom of the chart, shows this child's initial difficulties with sleep (does not sleep through most nights), digestion (has often been constipated, with poor appetite), focus/attention and self-regulation (unable to sustain attention, unable to shift out of hyperactive mode), social connection (could not connect with peers or teachers at school), tantrums (would have hour-plus meltdowns most afternoons), and touch sensitivity (head, face, ears, chest, tummy, fingers and/or toes painful to touch). In the two blank slots, this mother chose to follow potty training (multiple accidents most days and during the night) and picky eating (limited range of foods).

Now compare this same child at mid-year (darker line above). You can see at a glance that there have been significant improvements in each of the areas as compared to scores at the start date (lighter line below). The most improvement was in sleep, social connection, touch sensitivity, potty training and picky eating. It is quite typical that sleep is one of the first areas to improve for most children. As touch normalized and this child was more able to sense a wet diaper and feel the internal signals for her need to go to the bathroom, her potty training improved. The mother reported, "she began insisting we nighttime potty-train her and her daytime potty accidents completely stopped". This child's focus, attention, self-regulation and tantrums also showed improvement, just not as much as the other areas. It is typical that these areas take more time for improvements to unfold.

Using the example above, take a second look at the individual changes in each of your child's beginning and mid-year scores to understand in even greater detail what changes have taken place in the first six months. You may have already recognized some of these changes. Others may feel new to you. In another six months, at the end of the year, you'll complete this same chart a third time along with the checklists to see your progress over the year.

Next week, we will take a look at the other measure of progress you set out at the beginning – your own goals for yourself and your child. We will have you revisit those goals to see how many you have reached.

Congratulations on your good work!

Louisa and Linda

Sense and Self-Regulation Checklist

Name of child: _____   **Mid-Year Check Date:** _____

Please circle the response for each item that most accurately describes your child.

1. TACTILE = ORAL/TACTILE	Often	Sometimes	Rarely	Never
• Does not cry tears when hurt	3	2	1	0
• Doesn't notice if the diaper is wet or dirty	3	2	1	0
• Face washing is difficult	3	2	1	0
• Haircuts are difficult	3	2	1	0
• Refuses to wear a hat	3	2	1	0
• Prefers to wear a hat	3	2	1	0
• Cutting fingernails is difficult	3	2	1	0
• Prefers to wear one or two gloves	3	2	1	0
• Avoids wearing gloves	3	2	1	0
• Cutting toenails is difficult	3	2	1	0
• Will only wear certain footwear (e.g. loose shoes, no socks)	3	2	1	0
• Prefers to wear the same clothes day after day	3	2	1	0
• Will only wear certain clothes (e.g. no elastic, not tight, no tags, long or short sleeves)	3	2	1	0
• Cries tears when falls, scrapes skin, or gets hurt (scale is reversed on purpose)	0	1	2	3
• Head bangs on a hard surface	3	2	1	0
• Head bangs on a soft surface	3	2	1	0
• Avoids foods with certain textures	3	2	1	0
• Tooth brushing is difficult	3	2	1	0
• Mouths or chews objects	3	2	1	0
Self-regulation – Orientation/Attention/Self-soothing/Sleep	Often	Sometimes	Rarely	Never
• Has to be prompted to make eye contact when spoken to	3	2	1	0
• Seems not to notice when spoken to in a normal voice	3	2	1	0
• Does not respond to his/her name	3	2	1	0
• Does not notice or react when tapped on the back	3	2	1	0
• Does not roll over onto the back when asked	3	2	1	0
• Stares off into space	3	2	1	0
• Seems unaware when others are hurt	3	2	1	0
• Has difficulty calming him/herself when upset	3	2	1	0
• Gets upset or tantrums when asked to make a transition	3	2	1	0
• Has difficulty falling asleep at bedtime	3	2	1	0
• Has difficulty falling back asleep when awakens during the night	3	2	1	0
• Awakens very early and stays awake	3	2	1	0
• Has difficulty awakening in morning	3	2	1	0
• Makes little jokes (*Answer only if your child has language.*) (Scale is reversed on purpose)	0	1	2	3
SubTotal-pg 1: _____ [Sum of all columns]	☐	☐	☐	☐

Please circle the response for each item that most accurately describes your child.

2. SENSORY = VISION	Often	Sometimes	Rarely	Never
• Looks at objects out of sides of eyes	3	2	1	0
• Is bothered by certain lights	3	2	1	0

Self-regulation – Behavior: Irritability, Aggression, Self-injurious	Often	Sometimes	Rarely	Never
• Tantrums or meltdowns	3	2	1	0
(Tantrums last_____minutes, and occur_____times/day)				
• Cries easily when frustrated	3	2	1	0
• Hits or kicks others	3	2	1	0
• Scratches or pulls other's hair	3	2	1	0
• Bites others	3	2	1	0
• Throws things at others	3	2	1	0
• Pulls own hair (Where on the head?)	3	2	1	0
• Bites self (Which part of the body e.g. left thumb?)	3	2	1	0
• Hits self (Which part of the body?)_____	3	2	1	0
• Gets aggressive or 'hyper' with exposure to certain smells	3	2	1	0

3. SENSORY = HEARING	Often	Sometimes	Rarely	Never
• Reacts poorly to certain everyday noises	3	2	1	0
• Covers ears with certain sounds	3	2	1	0
• Reacts strongly when others cry loudly or scream	3	2	1	0
• Is startled by sudden noises	3	2	1	0

Self-regulation – Toilet training	Often	Sometimes	Rarely	Never
• Is dry at night (scale is reversed on purpose)	0	1	2	3
• Diaper is wet in the morning	3	2	1	0
• Wears a diaper during the day	3	2	1	0
• Is toilet trained (scale is reversed on purpose)	0	1	2	3

4. SENSORY = SMELL	Often	Sometimes	Rarely	Never
• Gags with certain smells	3	2	1	0

Self-regulation – Digestion	Often	Sometimes	Rarely	Never
• Will only eat familiar foods	3	2	1	0
• Does not seem to be interested in food	3	2	1	0
• Eats very few foods (five to ten items)	3	2	1	0
• Bowels are loose	3	2	1	0
• Bowel movements ("poops") are frequent (more than 3 per day)	3	2	1	0
• Requires regular use of laxative to avoid constipation	3	2	1	0
• Bowel movement ("poop") is hard and dry	3	2	1	0
• Has a bowel movement every other day	3	2	1	0
• Has a bowel movement twice a week	3	2	1	0
• Has a bowel movement once a week	3	2	1	0
• Bowel movements are often green	3	2	1	0

SubTotal pg 1: _____ SubTotal pg 2: _____   Total_____

Parent Stress Index

Name of child: _____   Mid-Year Check Date: _____

Please rate the following aspects of your child's <u>health according to how much stress it causes you and/or your family</u> by placing an X in the box that best describes your situation.	Stress Ratings				
	Not stressful	Sometimes creates stress	Often creates stress	Very stressful on a daily basis	So stressful sometimes we feel we can't cope
Your child's social development	0	1	2	3	5
Your child's ability to communicate	0	1	2	3	5
Tantrums/meltdowns	0	1	2	3	5
Aggressive behavior (siblings, peers)	0	1	2	3	5
Self-injurious behavior	0	1	2	3	5
Difficulty making transitions from one activity to another	0	1	2	3	5
Sleep problems	0	1	2	3	5
Your child's diet	0	1	2	3	5
Bowel problems (diarrhea, constipation)	0	1	2	3	5
Potty training	0	1	2	3	5
Not feeling close to your child	0	1	2	3	5
Concern for the future of your child being accepted by others	0	1	2	3	5
Concern for the future of your child living independently	0	1	2	3	5
Subtotal					
				Total	

Week 28

Checking in on Your Goals

Dear parents,

This week, we're going to take a look at another way to measure your progress by revisiting the goals that you set out when you began. At that time, we had you write down three things that you most wanted QST to change for your child so you would have a clear long-term picture of what you wanted to accomplish. We said that you'd come back to look at these goals in six months to see what progress you've made. So, let's take a look!

First, without looking back to your original goals, let's start right where you are today. Please list below the three changes or improvements that you most want to see for your child in the next six months:

1.
2.
3.

Now, please look back to Chapter 7 – Getting Started, on page 57 to find the original goals you wrote down six months ago and re-write them here:

1.
2.
3.

Now, let's compare your original goals with today's goals. Are they exactly the same? What are the differences? Do you see any of the changes you wanted to achieve when you started the QST routine? Have any of these challenges gotten easier? Do you see any small or big steps toward these first goals? Have you seen other changes you didn't anticipate? As you set new goals, it's easy to forget how your new targets rest on your previous achievements that you may have taken for granted. Please look carefully at these lists; they might help you to better see how far you have come.

As you head into the second half of this year-long journey, please keep all of these goals – those at the beginning and today's – close in mind. Goals tell us where we were, where we are and where we are headed. They motivate us along the way and give us a sense of confidence for the future. And don't forget to celebrate each of your victories, the small ones and the large ones, whenever you see them!

Next week, we will focus on some specific changes that you can look for in your child's behavior, movement and responses during QST. Noticing these small positive signs will help you to appreciate your successes with the treatment and show that change is truly underway.

Keep up the good work!

Louisa and Linda

Week 29

Changes and What They Mean

Dear parents,

This week, we want to point your attention to what, at first, may feel like small changes in your child's responses during QST. These are little, seemingly insignificant changes that you may not even notice, but they are big signs that you are achieving successful results with your daily treatment. Let's take a closer look at some of these easy-to-overlook signs. They are the early clues that important developmental changes are underway.

Head down. When your child can lie still on her belly without wiggling and put her head down during QST, you are getting a sign that her nervous system has begun to calm down. You will also see she starts to sleep better. When she can *remain* lying down for the entire treatment, it is a sign that her sense of touch overall is becoming normalized. These small behaviors mark especially important accomplishments because when the sense of touch is normalized, sensory and behavioral problems become less severe, and that paves the way for new strides in development.

Ears. Watch for the muscles of your child's neck becoming softer and more relaxed under your touch and see that you can touch her ears without triggering distress. Both are important signs that your child can start paying more attention to people's voices and can understand more of what you say to her. This will help her to focus her attention, understand and be able to follow instructions better.

Smiling. When your child can look at you and smile, especially during three particular QST movements – 'down the sides', 'ear to hand', and 'fingers' – she is showing you that she has accomplished the ability to do three separate things all together: turn toward you, make eye contact and listen. This sounds like a simple thing, but it is actually a complex physiological achievement that, in the absence of sensory or other problems, takes place automatically and seamlessly. When she starts to do these things with you more spontaneously, it is a signal that touch, hearing and vision have begun to integrate – and that's the starting point for all social development. Expect to see her paying attention to and interacting more with others.

Fingers. We've found that some children with sensory issues and low muscle tone often have poor awareness in their fingers and hands. It's as if they have gloves on! For others who are touch defensive, touching things or being touched on the hands and fingers feels really uncomfortable, painful and icky. When your child is more comfortable with her own fingers and open to having them touched during QST, she can begin to use them more freely. QST improves body awareness in general, and greater feeling and awareness in the fingers results in improvements in fine motor skills. Since our first language is gestural pointing, increased comfort in the fingers also signals that improvements in speech may follow. In our experience, many children show improvements in language as a result of QST, and even severely autistic and non-verbal children have acquired some speech. And, for those who don't acquire language, we have seen other improvements in development and behavior, along with a reduction in parent's stress levels.

Chest. Yawning or rubbing the eyes during the 'relax chest' movement is an excellent sign that your child will be more able to soothe and calm herself when she begins to feel upset. Children who show this sign have fewer meltdowns, and the distress tends to be shorter and milder. We've found that transitions will be easier too.

Belly. As her belly becomes more receptive to touch, you will find that your child will be open to eating more foods and that her bowels will become more regular. In fact, a growth spurt may be right around the corner.

Feet. As your child's feet become more comfortable – that is, as her response to your touch and her ability to experience enjoyable feeling in them improves – it signals that other gross motor skills are likely to improve as well.

If you haven't seen many or all of these signs yet, don't despair or give up. Each child's timing is different. The most important thing is that you know what signs to look for. So, refer back to this short list of little clues. Becoming aware of them will keep you from getting discouraged, and they'll keep you and your child on track to bigger changes ahead. And the best part about all of these changes is that as your child relaxes more into the daily routine, the overall level of physical and emotional stress is reduced for both of you. Children begin to ask for their QST, you both look forward to this special time together and your connection deepens. You'll feel like your batteries are recharged!

And that feels terrific!

Louisa and Linda

Week 30

"Ready to Learn"

A Mother's Story

Dear parents,

I committed to QST faithfully to help my 5-year-old son overcome sensory challenges, speech delay and overall self-regulation difficulties that were hindering him in every facet of life. Admittedly, I was not sure what to expect and was somewhat skeptical, but I decided an approach that I was able to do on my own that involved no use of medication was one I was more than willing to try. After all, what did we have to lose?

When we first began QST, my son was in a self-contained PreK class struggling academically, socially and with difficult behaviors. I'd often sit through IEP [individualized education plan] meetings and clinics with tears in my eyes as I would be told by teachers and therapists that most of the time my son cannot sit/focus and attend to a task – "he is not ready to learn." I can remember during the first few weeks we began QST, the avoidance and discomfort I saw in my son as we worked through the movements. It was so difficult to get through all the steps, and often one parent would be trying to complete the routine while the other held him just enough to get through it. Over time, his tolerance improved, and he was requesting his nightly QST, which he refers to as his "medicine". Indeed, we came to see QST was the 'medicine' our son had so desperately needed.

"The behaviorist…told us that the gains he has made are so remarkable that he no longer has any behavior plan in place."

Over the course of a six-month period with consistent QST, we started to see increased tolerance for nail clipping and haircuts, improved sleep, increased vocabulary and overall attention improvement. We weren't the only ones noticing significant changes in our son. I attended the first meeting for kindergarten with my son's teacher and therapists. Everyone around the table told us that my son had arrived at this school year "ready to learn"! The behaviorist that has worked with our son for a few years was in this meeting and told us that the gains he has made are so remarkable that he no longer has any behavior plan in place. His behaviors are no longer an issue, and now that he is self-regulated and ready to learn, his teacher and therapists can place the focus on academics, which our son is absorbing!

My son is now thriving in school, both socially and academically, as he has been able to be included in a variety of general education areas with his neurotypical peers, including gym, music, art, library and technology. He has come such a long way with QST, and I am truly so optimistic for our journey ahead. My advice to parents is to commit to QST and watch your child blossom. There may be times you question if QST is making any difference, but stay the course! Do not under-estimate the power of your own touch as it can be truly amazing.

All the best,

Diana

Mother of a 5-year-old

Week 31

Doing QST 6–7 Days A Week Versus 3–4 Days

Dear parents,

While a lot of research statistics can be dull and boring, sometimes they can give us an accurate picture of what things help and where the pitfalls lie. This week, we look at one segment of our own research data that gives a clear roadmap to what does and doesn't work and can provide you with a picture of how long you may need to continue the routine with your child.

Let's start with frequency. By now, you know how important it is to keep doing the daily QST routine 6–7 days a week. Most parents don't have too much trouble doing that for the first six months because their children's improvements are so obvious and satisfying. But many children in the second half of the year tend to settle down into a less dramatic pattern of growth. We have tracked the results in the first and second half of the year for parents who did the treatment 6–7 days a week and for those who dropped back to 3–4 days a week, and we found a big difference.

For the second half of the year, parents who continued QST 6–7 days a week could achieve an additional amount of new developmental skills equal to that which they saw in the first half of the year. So, for example, if their child improved 20% in language skills by mid-year, they could expect a 40% improvement by the end of the year. On the other hand, parents who dropped the frequency to 3–4 days a week in the second half of the year did not get the same results. While their children kept the gains they had made in the first half of the year, they did not continue to gain skills at the same rate as those who received QST every day. It was as if these children switched from catch-up mode to maintenance mode.

The other question that parents often ask, and that our research helps answer, is: how long will I have to keep up the daily schedule? The answer, according to our studies, has a lot to do with the child's age and their individual history of difficulties. By this point, your child's nervous system has been stuck in a well-established pattern of delayed growth for several years. Our studies have shown that for most children, you will need to give QST daily for at least half as long as that pattern has been in place. So, if your 3-year-old has had sensory problems since birth and you want to shift to a better path of continued improvements, you should expect to give QST for one-and-a-half years to accomplish the best sustainable results. If sensory problems began two years ago, you could plan for a daily routine for one year. Of course, each child is unique with unique difficulties but, in general, this rule holds.

However, there are also exceptions. Our research has shown that some children, specifically those who are higher functioning, continued to make good progress in the second half of the year with QST only 3–4 days a week. So, observe your child's progress closely, and know that the research clearly shows that there are greater benefits to be gained in the second half of the year and that there are always exceptions. Ultimately, you must make your decision based on what you know and sense about your child. If you decide to decrease frequency and you see old patterns emerge, it means that your child still needs the consistency of the daily routine for now. Continuing your daily QST is never a bad idea! QST is the most organizing, relaxing and energizing medicine we have. It boosts your child's nervous system in the direction of growth every single day.

All our best,
Louisa and Linda

Week 32

A Last Resort

A Mother's Story

Dear parents,

It was by chance that a friend referred me to my alma mater, and I made a distressed call to their Center for Autism and Early Childhood Mental Health. I was desperate and felt that this was a last resort to find help for my daughter. Not long after, I received a call from Linda, who kindly explained the program and met with me to introduce the QST technique. I was slightly guarded and questioned whether the method would be helpful, but I agreed to go ahead in the hopes that I was wrong.

This chance encounter turned out to be perfect timing. We were struggling with some really challenging behavior from my 4-year-old and had run the gamut of therapies, techniques and advice over the last few years. We were struggling mostly with behavior issues but also a sensory processing disorder. On a daily basis, my daughter would exhibit aggressive behavior, constant tantrums, picky eating, sleep problems, frequent potty accidents, anxiousness and defiance. I was hesitant to start this technique with my daughter, as it did necessitate a commitment to a daily routine. And at first, trying to get my spirited, high-energy daughter to slow down long enough to relax and absorb the treatment was difficult.

Initially, I was only able to get her to get through half of the steps of the routine. Certain parts, like my touching her fingers and toes, were incredibly bothersome. Some days, she refused altogether, and I let it go for those days. Some days, I couldn't handle doing it for her. However, we stuck to our promise and made QST a part of our nighttime routine. As days turned to weeks, my daughter started to learn the steps. She began to ask for QST randomly during the day when she felt she needed that connection with me. Not too long after, we fell into a good daily pattern. She started to enjoy getting the routine every day, and I enjoyed giving it to her. I have to say I didn't notice any changes at all over the course of the next few weeks and months. We still had rough days and weeks. However, after completing the two checklists and doing another set six months later, it was quite evident that we had started to see significant improvements and changes.

My picky eater started trying new foods with very little hesitation. She also began insisting we nighttime potty train her, and her daytime potty accidents completely stopped. She also slept through the night several times in her own bed, which she rarely did. Before, she had never acknowledged any sense of smell at all, but now her sense of smell has truly been completely opened. Now, almost a year later, she loves getting QST every day and looks forward to it.

A lot of the therapies we have tried (and we have tried many) have felt intrusive, even traumatizing to both of us and often caused my daughter to shut down completely. Doing QST is one of the most helpful therapies I've encountered. It's a gentle therapy where you work at your own pace with your child. This therapy has helped me reignite the reason I became a parent. When the times get tough, it's easy to pull away and disconnect from someone. Our bond is so much stronger now from doing this therapy, and I think the sheer skin-to-skin connection it has created all over again has helped our relationship tremendously.

At the end of the day, I think that is what all these children need. They are looking for that reconnection with the parent. Sometimes we get too focused on them becoming little independent adults and lose sight that they just want that real emotional, physical and mental connection with their parents. These techniques truly work, and we still incorporate it into our daily lives most nights of the week. It's something parents can do at home, it's affordable, it's calming, and it's been a life changer! It's my job to make sure my child feels peace within, and I am thankful every day, for we are truly blessed and grateful to have been introduced to QST and to Linda!

Julie
Mother of a 5-year-old

Extra Techniques – Weeks 33–42

Week 33

A Simple Technique to Stop Aggressive Behavior

Dear parents,

Aggressive behaviors can take many forms – pinching, hitting, kicking, biting and even spitting. These behaviors are usually triggered very quickly, sometimes with only a one- or two-second warning to tell you they are coming. And there is a very simple reason for this. It is not that your child is basically aggressive or willfully acting out. Her immature nervous system is easily tipped toward fight-or-flight, where she reacts instantly and automatically with survival behaviors that make it very difficult for her to learn how to deal appropriately with pain, threat or frustration. (see Chapter 1)

'Fight-or-flight' (our self-defense mode) and the aggressive behavior it can set off is commonly triggered by one of three things:

1. Touch feels painful.
2. Her personal space has been invaded too quickly.
3. Her wishes and needs were frustrated, or something that belongs to her has been taken away.

These are not easy things to deal with. Children aren't born knowing appropriate behavior; they have to learn it from their parents. When a child becomes aggressive, parents need to first stop the behavior in a way that helps guide her out of the fight-or-flight stress mode that she is in. The next step is to demonstrate how to respond appropriately. That can only be achieved when she is in a calm and receptive mode.

That is where the *other* survival mechanism comes into play, the relax-and-relate mode. This is the mode that dials down the fight-flight part of the brain and makes your child receptive to connecting with you. It also activates the part of the brain responsible for all of the self-regulation abilities that we have been talking about so far – sleep, self-soothing and paying attention. It's the place where all learning begins. When all goes well, a child's brain is hard-wired to respond to a parent's attuned, reassuring touch with a relaxation response. This is the brain state needed to learn to re-direct stress behaviors into the more developmentally appropriate behaviors that you show her. Your QST helps to normalize your child's touch and sensory reactivity so that your daily

DOI: 10.4324/9781003360421-22

touch treatment can activate and strengthen the relax-and-relate mode on a regular and repeated basis. Here are the simple – but effective – steps to take when these stress behaviors arise.

Hitting or pinching. Immediately reach out and firmly but gently squeeze the hand that pinched or hit and say in a *firm but loving voice*, "No hitting [pinching]. Gentle hands." It will probably surprise your child, but your kind and firm pressure will re-focus her awareness back into her body and help to switch her brain into receptive mode. Then she can hear you. Continue firm pressure until you feel her hands relax.

Kicking. The moment your child kicks, take both feet (or legs) firmly in your hands, squeeze them gently but firmly and say in a resolute but calmly loving voice, "No kicking. Gentle feet". If she is lying down, put firm but gentle pressure above both knees and say the same thing. Continue until she relaxes her feet and legs.

Biting or spitting. Firmly press down on both shoulders at the same time, then firmly, gently and slowly squeeze down the arms to the hands while saying in a firm but calmly loving voice, "No biting [spitting]. Gentle." Repeat this several times, holding her hands lovingly but firmly in yours.

Your first impulse when you see aggressive behavior will be to try to stop it. But you can't stop the behavior until you first help your child back to relax-relate mode. So, *your first step is to calm yourself.* And remember, your child's behavior is not willful, it is an automatically triggered response. *Your child does not like her distressful behavior any more than you do.*

This is key!

Your face, voice and touch must convey safety, not threat. These tips won't work if you are upset, your voice is raised or your face shows anger or a hint of threat. They also won't work if you wait to do these things 5 or 10 minutes later. You must respond the moment the behavior begins. Remaining calm and resolute in the moment is not always easy, but it is absolutely necessary to stop the challenging behavior.

Usually, these behaviors will stop immediately, and if your child is verbal, then you can talk with her about what happened and encourage her to use her words instead. For the less verbal child, you may also say, "When we are frustrated, we use our words." If she is non-verbal, it is often enough to just stop the behavior.

While the frequency of these behaviors tends to drop quickly, you may need to repeat these actions whenever the behavior recurs. Your resolute tone of voice and calm expression are key elements for success because your child's nervous system is exquisitely tuned to even the slightest signal of threat from voices and faces. Achieving this is not always easy in the heat of the moment, especially if you are hurt, but the more you experience how you can help your child find the receptive mode, the easier it will be. Once you get the hang of it, we think it will work well for you. It's one of the best ways to help your child learn the kind of behavior you both are more comfortable with.

Wishing you the best of luck,

Louisa and Linda

Week 34

Getting Your Child out of Defense Mode

Reflections From a QST Master Trainer

Dear parents,

Sometimes nothing will do – your child is so, so sensitive and there is no way that you can touch her. She might scream, kick or even bite and push you away so you won't be able to touch her at all. This happens when children are overwhelmed, and while this overwhelm may happen for all sorts of reasons, it primarily happens because they are stuck in defense mode. As a parent, you know perfectly well what overwhelms your child. And your instincts will tell you to protect her at whatever cost. To do that, you may try to micromanage her environment. But this is a never-ending story, one that will leave you frustrated, exhausted and disappointed. I know, I felt like that when my children got overwhelmed and I tried to protect them from every little influence or evil that could happen to them.

Since then, I found a better way to deal with a child that is so overwhelmed that she is stuck in fight or flight. The best way to help is to get her back into her body and help her to ground. That's because our sense of safety is in the body. So here is what you do: Stand behind your child and apply deep pressure on her shoulders in a slow rhythmic way. The more she is agitated, the more slowly and deep the pressure you should apply. Sometimes her overwhelm is so great that the pressure she needs to calm her nervous system down and get her back into her body can feel especially strong or more intense than how you commonly press. Calmly lean into your child's shoulders with your whole body with the intention to ground, *not* control her. (The goal is to provide a feeling of safe 'containment', not restraint.) Continue the deep pressure until she calms. Dads can be particularly good with this technique.

This is a technique I have found that works really well when you are calm and grounded yourself. I hope this little technique will help you help your child on her healing journey.

I wish you the best of luck.

Warmly,

Sabine Baeyens

QST Master Trainer

Amsterdam, Netherlands

www.qsti.org/master-trainers/

Week 35

Points From Chinese Medicine That Help the Brain

Dear parents,

Over 3000 years ago, Chinese medicine practitioners developed a detailed map of the energy flow in the body, including the network of points and channels that carry that flow. This week, we'll show you three of those important energy points that are key to your effectiveness with QST. You've been using these points in your daily routine, but now we'll show you how focusing your attention and intention on them will enhance your effectiveness and help integrate the sensory information your child's brain is receiving. Let's look at these three key energy points:

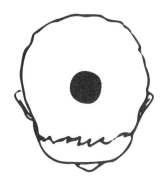

The center point at the top of the head. Both the 'down the back' and 'down the sides' movements start at this point, the soft spot at the center top of the head. This is a particularly important master point in Chinese medicine because of its capacity to regulate the body's active, outward energies (yang energy). This point brings a child's awareness to her body and opens the senses to her immediate surroundings.

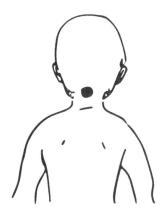

Point at the base of head/neck. Both of the 'down the back' movements pass over this point where the head and neck meet at the base of the skull. This point activates your child's attention. It helps her coordinate three key activities: turning to face you, focusing her eyes on your face and tuning her ears to your voice. These are three essential components of social attention that, when integrated, open a pathway to learn social, emotional and language skills.

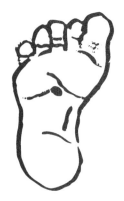

Point at the bottom of the foot. The last movement, 'nourish and integrate – rhythmic wave', starts with either your thumbs or the palms of your hands on this point on the bottom of the feet. It is the point where the body connects to the earth when standing and the place we push off from when walking. The rhythmical rocking movement you create by pressing on this spot as the final movement in the QST routine sends a wave of restful energy through the body and up to the brain that helps the brain integrate all the sensory information involved in upright movement.

Over the next two weeks, we will show you how to use these points in extra techniques. You can use them at any time throughout the day when your child may need extra support to calm down hyperactive energies and heightened stressful emotions or to simply re-focus her attention.

Best wishes,
Louisa and Linda

Week 36

The Easy Button

Dear parents,

In the next two weeks, we will share two techniques that use the key energy points we talked about last week. You've already been using these points in your daily QST. Now we'll show you how to use them at any point, anywhere during the day when your child needs additional support. This week's 'easy button' helps bring regulation when your child's nervous system is on hyper-alert, while next week's 'face-me button' helps to organize focus and attention. We call these two touch techniques 'buttons' because they are like having a special button that helps your child's body regulate to a calmer state. But this is not a button that you 'push' as a way of control. It's a special point from Chinese medicine that gives you access to deliver your touch signals to just the right place, and in just the right way, to turn off the stress response and activate the regulating influence of the relax-relate mode.

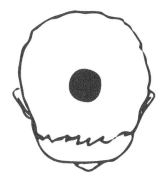

Settling the stress. What we call the 'easy button' is simply that center point on the top of the head where we start the 'down the back' movement. This is that important master point in Chinese medicine and is involved in regulating energy throughout the body, opening the senses to our immediate surroundings and bringing bodily awareness.

This spot is especially effective when your child's stress response is escalating and you want to help calm her nervous system. It can also be quite effective for children who toe walk. Patting the 'easy button' will often help your child to settle down on to her heels. As with every movement in QST, the key is observing your child's response and adjusting your technique to what works best to guide her to a calm, attentive, more comfortable place.

Let's look at a good example from one mother who reported how she used it with her agitated son. She was waiting for a bus with her son who was bouncing up and down and becoming increasingly hyper. Instead of getting caught up in his intensifying energy or becoming reactive to him, she remembered the 'easy button' and began patting that spot on the top of his head. Within a minute, he calmed down and stood still beside her until the bus came. She was amazed at the result and that there was something she could actually do to connect with her son and help him regulate during times when his distress was increasing.

When using the 'easy button', start with the same cupped, relaxed hand that you use in the 'down the back' movement in the daily routine. A medium tapping speed sometimes works best. At other times, a slow pulsing pressure is better. The next time your child's nervous energy starts to wind up, use the speed and pressure that helps most to calm the stress – but remember, your first job is to bring your attention to your own relaxed exhale and to find a calm and relaxed place from which to begin. Then you can best help your child find hers.

All our best,
Louisa and Linda

Week 37

The Face-Me Button

Dear parents,

This week, we share a second technique you can use any time that your child's nervous system is in distress mode, making it difficult for her to focus her attention, or if she needs extra help to calmly engage with you.

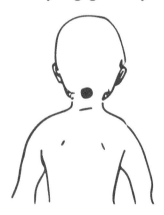

Helping to focus attention. This second spot, the 'face-me button' is located at the bottom ridge of the skull/top of the spine, where your child's head meets her neck. You have already been tapping into this area while doing the 'down the back' movement. In Chinese medicine, this is an important energy point for integrating the brain, tongue and speech. It connects directly to the part of the brain that activates your child's attention and her natural instinct to face you when you call her name. That ability to face others and respond when your name is called is an important skill that every child needs for school. But answering to your name, which involves facing the person and making eye contact, is very stimulating to the nervous system, making what would appear to be an easy task quite difficult for a child in fight-or-flight or shut-down mode. Using this technique will help her build and strengthen this skill.

If your child is involved in something else and you want her to face you and pay attention, here is what you do once you are relaxed: sit or stand beside her at eye level and start patting with the center of your cupped hand over this spot. The key is to pat at a pace that gives your child time to register and calm to your touch. After you have patted a few times, call her name. At first, your child will need the patting on this spot to face you as you call her. Once you've helped her nervous system get into the relax-relate mode, a child's natural response is to turn toward you and be ready for conversation. Over time, you will build and strengthen her own capacity to engage with you without the patting first.

Two great things about both the 'easy button' from last week and this week's 'face-me button' are that they use the same principles as the QST protocol that you are already using and, most importantly, they work! We hope that you will find them to be effective tools that bring the calming benefits of the routine into everyday life. Our goal is to begin with your daily routine and end with an overall ability to self-regulate throughout the entire day. And if you should discover any other techniques that work for you, please let us know!

All our best,

Louisa and Linda

Week 38

Making Transitions Easier

Dear parents,

If you child is having difficulties making transitions, now is a good time to try this additional technique. She is ready for this help because she is used to the routine and can calm down much more quickly in response to your touch and your calm voice. Most importantly, you are now able to trigger the self-soothing response (rubbing eyes, yawning) when doing the 'relax chest' movement and her tantrums are fewer, shorter and less intense.

The inability to make smooth transitions is one of the hallmarks of an immature sensory nervous system. This can be something as simple as an inability to move from one activity to another without a meltdown or not stopping her play to come to dinner. Although she enjoys family dinners, she still resists your request. Why? Because change isn't easy, and to make a smooth transition, she has to first be able to listen and pay attention to what is expected. She also needs to remain calm and open when she gives up one thing and starts the next. That is where she needs your extra support.

At times like these, parents can feel frustrated and helpless. They may begin to bargain, bribe or use distractions to get their child to cooperate through the transition. "If you come with me to pick up your sister, I'll give you a candy bar." But bribing, bargaining and distractions are only temporary solutions to a deeper problem. Your child needs to learn to navigate transitions smoothly because, on the road ahead, life is going to require that she master this basic skill.

We offer a simple and effective technique that you can use to help her make these transitions, but *it will only work once you've been able to trigger the self-soothing response* in the 'relax chest' movement. In other words, she has to have first learned to relax with pressure on her chest. Here again you use your touch to focus her attention and help her calm. Let's say your child is watching TV and you want her to come to the dinner table. Here's what you do:

1. **Make a connection with touch.** Sit next to her, without saying anything. Place one hand on the front of her chest and the other hand on her back directly behind her chest. Make a firm and gentle connection.
2. **Give the instruction.** When you feel that she has noticed you, tell her: "It's time to come and eat dinner."

3. **Repeat and offer help.** If she doesn't respond or start to move on her own, repeat, "It's time to come and eat dinner" and ask if she needs help.
4. **Give physical guidance.** If she still doesn't respond, keep a steady hold (back and front) on her chest and guide her upright saying, "Let's go and eat dinner." Walk next to her holding her chest between your hands until she sees the dinner table and her chair. At that point, she should be able to complete the transition and sit down in her chair for dinner.
5. **For a video example**, see the *Making Transitions Easier* online resource (Appendix H, page 221).

This may sound overly simple, but it can be very effective, and you'll be surprised how much better it works than just telling her to come to dinner. Most children basically like to eat, but change can be very difficult and threatening. When you place pressure on her chest and her back, you re-trigger the self-soothing response that you have been developing and strengthening over these many weeks. That extra support helps her to feel calm while she switches from doing one thing and transitions to the next. With time, you'll be able to achieve the same result with only a firm and gentle hand on the middle of her back.

Have fun with this!

Louisa and Linda

Week 39

Adapting to My Child's Needs

A Mother's Story

Note from Linda and Louisa: This mother's story is a beautiful example of finding a way to adapt the daily routine to the specific sensory needs of her child in the moment. Her daughter 'knew' her body needed to jump. Mom reframed the behavior not as 'bad behavior', but as a cue that her daughter needed that active movement to process the feelings and sensations in her body at that moment. Instead of becoming frustrated and trying to control and eliminate this behavior, this mother adapted by using the short rest period to do the QST movements, bringing order and rhythm to her daughter's natural drive for movement. And an equally important lesson from this mother was the way that she also listened to her own body and adapted to the needs of her own well-being.

Dear fellow parents,

We've experienced so many benefits from the QST protocol that I quickly became dedicated to it. We went three weeks without missing a night (which feels like a small miracle)! And then one night, we were behind schedule, I had a headache and I was exhausted. My daughter was looking forward to it, and I know how beneficial it is to have a consistent and daily routine. So even though I felt burned out, I started to power through . . . something that is a bit of a habit for me. I could feel myself getting edgy and impatient, and then I remembered the permission I had been given to skip a night if I wasn't feeling well or able to feel calm enough to create a supportive experience. So, after some internal struggle, I looked my daughter in the eyes and while holding her hand I said, "I'm so sorry. I really look forward to this. This time with you is so special to me, but we are running out of time and I'm exhausted, so we can't do the whole thing tonight." I added, "I'm sorry if you are disappointed. Instead you can pick your three favorite movements and maybe we can do more during the day tomorrow."

The next two things amazed me! First, she amazed me by handling the disappointment so well. This is *not* a typical experience in our household. Then, the next day when we did do more of the movements as I had promised, I surprised myself! Before her quiet time, she had loads of energy – something that *is* a typical experience in our household – and something that usually makes me feel frustrated as I try to cultivate calm during 'quiet time'. My daughter started to jump on the bed and wanted me to watch her and count her jumps. This time, instead of resisting her activity, I surprised myself by using her little rest periods to do QST. She jumped five times, while I counted aloud. Then she fell down and rested for one second. She got up and jumped ten times while I counted, and then she fell down and rested for one second. I decided to do one of the QST movements during every rest period. She absolutely adored this experience! She jumped and jumped and then she laid down for a few minutes between the exertions. We went through each of the 12 movements in her jumping breaks. Once again, she directed me and we enjoyed a completely new way to share the QST routine during the day. Normally clingy, my daughter was now able to calmly separate and go about her independent playtime.

I continue to learn so much from this process. Thank you!

Asha

Mother of a 7-year-old

Week 40

Release of Emotions During QST

During QST one day, my son just started sobbing. If I hadn't been warned about this I definitely would have stopped right then! But I kept doing what I was doing and the sobbing stopped just as quickly as it had started. He didn't seem to really even notice he had been sobbing. It felt like something deep inside that needed to come out, came out.

Mother of a 5-year-old

Dear parents,

As a parent, you are aware of the unpleasant emotions that can arise in you when you encounter challenging behaviors. These emotions, often hard to admit or talk about, include anger, sadness, grief, frustration and sometimes even fury. Children feel exactly the same emotions, and they absorb all of their family's feelings as well. Often unable to express, process or even understand their emotions, they tend to hold onto them, and these feelings can get 'stuck' in their bodies. You can see the same thing in adults who, when under stress, may have chronic headaches or stomachaches.

As your child learns the relaxation response in the daily QST routine, emotions that may have been stored away in the muscles and tissues may be released. Don't be surprised if your child suddenly expresses a burst of strong or unexpected feelings. You'll find that these emotional bubbles most often happen after you've been doing QST for a few months and as new pathways for energy and relaxation have had a chance to integrate. When these emotions first bubble up it can be difficult, even scary, for parents to see. When a child suddenly dissolves into a sorrowful sob, it's natural for a parent to stop what they are doing because they are afraid that they are hurting their child. But don't stop. This is exactly the place you can be of most help with your skilled touch and tender listening, giving the message that it is okay to feel those feelings. Your calm and reassuring presence creates a safe cocoon in which to experience these feelings without shutting them down prematurely.

When these emotional bubbles pop up, they are a very positive sign because they show that your child is now able to first feel and then release old and painful feelings. When these feelings arise, just do the same thing you've been doing to release tight muscles and energy blockages in the body; that is, use your skilled touch to help your child through the experience. Next week, we will show you how to do this so you won't be afraid or run away from the feelings at these important moments. And you will help your child free blocked emotional energy so that it can be expressed in more mature and related ways.

Best wishes,
Louisa and Linda

Week 41

Emotional Bubbles – How to Help

While doing the chest movement I noticed my son's chin start to quiver, then he erupted in tears, calling out Sharon, Sharon. I was shocked. This is the name of his teacher's aide who left his class recently for maternity leave. I gathered myself when I realized what these tears meant, rested my hands on his chest and told him it was okay to be sad that Sharon was gone. That her new baby needed her now and she was safe. His tears flowed for a little bit as he repeated her name, then just as quickly, his tears dried, he took a big deep breath and a smile came across his face as if the sun just came out. I'm still amazed!

Mother of a 4-year-old

Dear parents,

Last week, we talked about how the release of emotional bubbles can open the door to positive change and growth. This week, let's look more closely at what to watch for and what to do when they arise. The first and most important thing is to resist your natural instinct to stop the treatment. Continue with the part of the routine that you are doing when the emotion bubbles up. Many parents find this a very hard thing to do. Naturally, you want to stop and comfort your child! But what your child really needs at these moments is for you to continue working on that area, reassuring her with your calm touch and telling her that she is safe to feel these feelings and that you will be there with her. Remain focused on this area, but slow your movements down; you can even stop there with your hands resting in place if she needs a quiet moment. Reassure her that she is okay until the emotions have completely released. They usually pass very quickly once the feelings are out. Try to be matter-of-fact while lovingly reassuring your child with your warm and calm voice, "You're okay, you're okay", as she releases the painful feelings and the tears subside. Adults find it hard to believe how quickly their child's emotions will pass because as adults, our emotions can linger on and on. But for children, it's 'feel it and be done with it'. That's why we call them 'bubbles' – the emotions literally bubble to the surface, pop and are usually gone just as quickly.

Some emotions occur more commonly within different body areas and during specific QST movements, so let's take a look at some very specific types of feelings and where they commonly come up. For example, your child may release sorrow or grief when doing the 'relax chest' movement. Here you can see a quivering chin, a few tears or even a heart-wrenching sob with many tears. A second common area for emotional release is the belly, where fear, shock and even anger are the more typical emotions that come out. Again, don't be alarmed or feel you have to stop. Continue doing the movement, but slow it down and leave room for the feelings to be felt. It is your calm, quiet and reassuring voice that allows your child to feel safe and to fully feel, then release, these feelings. Once the emotion is out, continue with the rest of the routine as usual.

When emotions like these come up, it means that areas of the body holding these feelings are opening up and healing. It's a wonderful sign that you have made progress and have opened a path for change and growth. We have seen very positive improvements in a child's behavior following such releases. You will find, for example, that the child who had been holding tension may experience greater ease and relaxation, while the fearful child may now be more receptive to new situations. Not every child has these emotional releases, but many do. It's important for you to know about and be ready for them. Then, rather than withdrawing or trying to make the feelings go away, you can help your child work through them. Knowing what to anticipate and what to do prepares you to respond in the most helpful way when these strong emotions bubble up.

Best wishes,

Louisa and Linda

Week 42

Getting Through Emotionally Hard Times

A Parent's Story

Dear fellow parents,

I'm so grateful for Qigong and to have this chance to share with other parents just how much it has helped my daughter and me through some really hard times in our family. To make a long story short, my husband and I divorced when Jilia was just a year old. Unfortunately, it was one of those horrible, devastating divorces that involved a really vicious custody battle that lasted for years. My precious daughter, who was already struggling with wide-ranging symptoms, bore the brunt of the conflict, a long, drawn-out custody battle and relentless manipulation by the very adults who were supposed to be her source of security and comfort. She even ended up being diagnosed with PTSD as a result. My heart just breaks when I consider what we went through during those years. We were both pretty broken.

A friend told me about Qigong Sensory Treatment and told me that Jilia and I really needed it! I believed her. She gave me the book and videos, and I learned the routine and started doing it every single day, except when Jilia was at her father's. At first, her body was pretty rigid through most of the movements, especially in her neck and shoulders. Her fingers and toes were super sensitive. Her toes were so painful I could hardly touch them. But after only a few days, she was much more receptive to the whole routine. Her entire body seemed more relaxed. I remember one day early on, Jilia wanted to watch the videos of Dr. Silva giving the treatment, the ones that come with the book. I thought for sure she'd lose interest after five minutes, but she was entranced for the full 30 minutes! I think she especially liked watching the kids on the video getting QST.

One thing that really bothered me at first is that Jilia would cry and become very emotional, especially with the feet, and then after with the chest and belly. I mean, it was really heart-wrenching crying, and it was hard to watch and to not stop the movements, I have to admit. I would sometimes cry myself, but I kept on, doing the routine and telling her, "You're okay, Jilia, you're okay", like the book says to do. It was so hard! There was so much going on for her emotionally, but QST helped her release a lot of grief and pain that she hadn't felt safe to release any other way. And she kept asking for it every day, so she knew on some level that it was helping her.

There was also a time when she had 'night terrors' and would wake up in a panic screaming, "Momma! Where are you? Don't leave me!" over and over again. It was very disturbing. One night, I felt an instinct to do QST with her in that moment. Her response was instant, and she calmed right down, took huge deep breaths and fell fast asleep! There was a lot going on for me emotionally too during this time. Sometimes I felt so much shame that she wasn't with me more and I was always an emotional mess when she had to leave to go to her dad's.

Within a few months, Jilia was so much more relaxed and her whole body would just 'let go' the minute we started. She would unconsciously sigh, and as the giver of the QST, I felt much more confident and able to feel her energy and responses and offer her love, feeling and healthy energy. There is a very special bonding that happens that is very intimate between us. Jilia says she likes being touched by her momma, that it makes her feel good and calm. We're both healing.

One huge physical difference was in her swimming. It was as if something finally connected her body and mind. One day I was moved to tears watching her glide across the pool in freestyle. She had never swum that well, so in sync with stroke, body placement in the water, breathing, strength. She was beautiful! Another time, she had to have two teeth extracted and nearly flipped out in the dentist chair. I quietly did QST on her lower limbs as she lay in the chair, and whispered to her that I was helping her to ground in our 'special' way with love and breath. She knew what I was doing, and she settled down while the dentist worked on her.

A year into QST, Jilia had overcome a lot of her anxiety and fears and was having so many successes on so many levels in school, in sports and in her own feelings and emotions. Three years into it, I was overcome with gratitude and joy that she had come through a long emotionally exhausting time and is happy, confident and independent. We're now five years in, and yes, we still do Qigong. We both love it, and it helps both of us feel calm and centered. Qigong is and has been amazing for Jilia; it has totally supported her recovery from trauma and PTSD and helped her learn many tools she still incorporates today as coping skills when the world and its energies drain her completely. We both learned so much; I am so grateful that I learned to give Jilia this treatment, and I hope other parents love this as much as we do.

Yours truly,

Jilia's Mom

QST for Specific Needs – Weeks 43–50

Week 43

Stuck in Stress Mode

Dear parents,

Typically around the age of two, children start to understand that they are their own person. What used to be labeled the 'terrible two's' we've now come to understand as stress behavior. Assertive behavior is actually quite natural at this stage. But for children with immature nervous systems, their sense of confusion with sensory inputs can make it hard to mature and transition out of this phase. In fact, they can easily get stuck and for some children this phase can persist when they are 3, 4, 5 or more years old.

Saying "no" during this phase is your child's way of saying he wants to do everything for himself and asserting himself in this way can actually give him pleasure. And once he learns he can say no, he wants to practice it. We once counted 17 'no's' during a single conversation with a child. These new feelings of self-awareness, self-assertion and learning how to do for oneself are the keys to healthy independence and are good signs of developmental progress! But like most new things that a child learns, like playing with a new toy or re-hearing a bedtime story, they want to practice by doing it again and again and again, and this is where the 'terrible' part comes in. The behavior can be exhausting, leading some parents to misinterpret it as anger or willful defiance.

At this stage, children can benefit from a combination of freedom and a choice of options mixed with clear boundaries and limits. This sounds more complicated than it seems! For example, when your child begins to repeatedly say "No!", it can help to shift – offer him some options. Choices help, because this stage is not only about achieving autonomy; it's about learning to have more freedom, make decisions and stay safe – it's about options, rules and limits. So, when his behavior gets stuck or repetitive, offer your child two options. But be sure to make those choices limited and firm because too much freedom, too many choices and too loose boundaries can be frightening and confusing, leading to even more acting out.

Present two choices and make it clear that more are *not* an option. Offer the options firmly. For example, if he says "no" to putting his sweater on, ask – does he want to put his sweater on himself or does he want you to help him? He will almost always make a choice because that is what he really wants – to have a say in what happens! There is almost always something about the situation where you can offer a choice. But giving him a say doesn't mean

DOI: 10.4324/9781003360421-23

putting him in control. Sometimes parents have been so traumatized by their child's tantrums that they are afraid to set limits with their child and stick to them. Don't be afraid. Place firm limits on his choices so he can learn that he has some autonomy and that the options you give him will keep him safe.

All of this is especially important for children struggling with sensory difficulties. If you find that your 3- or 4- or 5-year-old is still stuck in this stage, don't be flummoxed. Remember that with QST, you are helping your child learn to self-regulate, bond and calm the very triggers that got his behavior stuck in a repetitive cycle in the first place. That helps to make your child even more receptive to your combination of choices, with limits. So you won't have to worry about teaching your 5-year-old those skills that a 2-year-old should have! For most older children, this phase usually doesn't last as long (with daily QST, possibly only a few weeks) as it would for a typical 2-year-old. By setting these clear boundaries and helping him to self-regulate, you help him understand the difference between something he has an option about and something that is not his decision. And, with your patience and suitable choices, he will catch up quickly and grow out of this stage, no matter what his age. He'll learn to trust you to give him the freedom he can handle and keep him safe the rest of the time. Then he'll be on to the next phase of development.

Good work!

Linda and Louisa

Week 44

Reframing the Need for Control

Dear parents,

Last week we talked about the best way to deal with a child stuck in the stress mode (what used to be called the 'terrible two's') – offering limited choices and setting appropriate rules and limits. This week, we're going to look at another fairly common phase of childhood, dealing with a child who is stuck in what used to be labeled the 'controlling four's', which we reframe as the need for predictability. This phase typically occurs around age four. Children start making the rules for the family and the family obeys. For example, the child doesn't want to go out to breakfast so the family doesn't go. Or the child doesn't want the mother to pay attention to anyone else, so the mother stays away from others whenever the child is around. It's very easy for parents to get drawn into a spiraling cycle where they essentially obey the child to avoid explosive conflicts. But when this occurs, the authority in the household has turned upside down, leaving the child with a feeling that his parents can't be counted on to set boundaries for safe and appropriate behavior. Without good rules or limits, he takes control as his only way to feel safe, and in the end, nobody is happy.

The way to change the situation is to first change the lens. Instead of seeing these as controlling misbehaviors, let's look at what may be causing the stress behavior that is driving the need to control. All of us make sense of the world by making predictions based on previous experiences. But for children with immature or disorganized sensory inputs, that process can become jumbled in their minds, leading to an ongoing stress response that fuels the need to create a safe, unchanging and predictable world. So, it is important to establish and then confidently and compassionately maintain fair, consistent boundaries and limits so that your child will feel that he has an anchor and a guide to see him through this age's emotional storms. Children need to know that *it is your job* as his parent to keep him safe. That means you will set fair rules and limits and that you'll enforce them.

As you begin, be alert to your own possible feelings of guilt around taking control (see Chapter 5) and try to remember that compassionate boundaries and structure are what your child needs to get through this phase. You will find that QST will be your assistant during this time. The daily routine will help to establish your child's trust that you can take charge while maintaining safe boundaries that will give him a sense of well-being. He will experience a growing sense of safety in his body, along with an increasing ability to regulate his emotions. Then, with the security of new self-control, he will no longer need to control others.

But be prepared for a few tantrums as you get through the adjustment period. Remember, at the outset, he will test your resolve to make sure he can count on you to be consistent. Just remember that while he is initially resisting you, he is also testing you, hungry for your compassionate resolve. This transition period, while not always easy, should not take more than a few days, especially when both parents work together and support the new plan. When that phase is completed, the entire family will breathe a sigh of relief and your child will feel more secure.

Good job!

Linda and Louisa

Week 45

What to Do About Regression

Dear parents,

All children have regressions. When we regress emotionally or behaviorally, we fall back to an earlier means of coping with the problem at hand. Children don't develop in a straight line. It's more of a zig zag pattern. They learn new skills by repeatedly 'practicing' each day through play and movement, and they feel exuberant at their new accomplishments. But when they encounter a novel problem or situation that is too much for the coping skills they've developed to date, they can get overwhelmed and fall back on forms of coping that they'd relied on at an earlier stage, like crying, freezing or running away. This is all a normal part of development.

Regressions simply mean a child is having trouble dealing with his life at that moment. Depending on the cause, regression can be small or big, lasting a few days or a few weeks. Small regressions can happen if a child gets too tired, hungry or stressed. In these cases, a little rest, a good meal, downtime and a good night's sleep are usually all that's needed. Bigger regressions happen in response to life's bigger changes and losses and let us know that our child needs more ongoing emotional support and downtime to regroup and integrate. As long as parents catch on to the reasons for the regression and provide the extra support needed, the regressions don't need to spiral out of hand. It also helps to remember that most regressions are temporary and there are some specific things you can do with QST that can help! So, let's take a look at some common signs that you might see and how to respond.

Growth spurt. Sometimes, just before or after a big growth spurt or developmental step, your child will have a regression. This is a normal and expectable part of development. Your child's behavior can revert to what feels like old patterns as his system re-organizes and integrates at a new level. Increase your daily QST routine to twice a day and be sure to spend lots of time on Movement 2 on the chest for extra regulating support. Your child will often need more of the slower, deeper pressing movements during these times.

Illness. Regressions are especially common after an illness or injury as your child struggles to deal with the changes in his body. Be patient. You may have to change your QST technique, patting more to clear out the toxins from the illness or the blocked circulation from an injury and then pressing to strengthen again. So, just continue your daily QST and in a few days – or a few weeks in some cases – your child will recover from the illness and the regression it caused. You could even give QST more than once a day to support him in his recovery.

Toxins. Regression can also be the result of toxins from something a child eats or exposure to fumes from magic markers, solvents or other environmental chemicals. When you follow some basic simple steps with regard to your child's diet – eliminating junk food, foods containing red dyes, MSG and environmental toxins in your home – it can result in dramatic improvements. Doing QST twice a day during this time will also help move these toxins out of your child's body, and toxic reactions will pass within a few days once the offending substance is removed (see also *Chapter 12 – Optimizing Diet, Nutrition and Daily Routines*).

Emotions. QST helps children become more aware of themselves and their emotions. But as that growing awareness happens, they often have to process some difficult emotions they haven't previously been in touch with but that have been held or 'stored' in the muscles and tissues of the body. It can cause an emotional reaction in your child that you are not used to or haven't seen before. This isn't a regression, but a sign of progress! Give your child time, patience and emotional support. During the daily routine, watch carefully to see where he needs more nurturing or strengthening (pressing) and where he needs help clearing out (patting). This can be a challenging few weeks, but keep up the daily QST routine and he will work through the backlog of emotion and be much better in touch with and able to process emotions as they come up in the future (see also *Week 40 – Release of Emotions* and *Week 41 – Emotional Bubbles – How to Help*).

Temporary ups and downs of life. If after considering this list of possible causes of regression you still don't know why your child is showing regressive symptoms, you can assume that he is stressed in some way. Do lots of Movement 2 on the chest; it will help his nervous system to calm down and process the stress. Your confident, consistent and compassionate support will help him transition through the normal ups and downs of life.

Bigger life changes. Children with sensory problems are no different from any other child. They can regress in response to all the usual life changes and losses that would cause any young child to regress – trouble in school, change to a new school or a new class, changes at home, illness in the family, loss of a caregiver, etc. You'll want to be particularly dedicated to continuing QST during these times. The soothing connection with you, through your touch and your own calm, will quiet his nervous system and support him while he processes the change or loss. It will give you some healing intimate time with your child. It is also a time to make sure he is getting enough sleep and eating well. This is just as important for parents too!

So, if you do encounter some of these signs of regression, you now understand that they can be periods of normal development that just *feel* like regression and you can be confident that the daily QST routine and specific QST extra techniques that you have learned (see *Extra Techniques in Weeks 33–42*) will help you and your child move successfully through any difficult period.

Warmest wishes,

Louisa and Linda

Week 46

Widening Social Circles (Parents – Siblings – Grandparents – Friends)

Dear parents,

While we have looked at a number of positive changes that result from using QST, perhaps the most obvious but often unrecognized one has to do with expanding a child's social circle. Over the years, we've noticed that with QST, children who have had constricted social circles are able to widen those connections in a predictable and normative way and catch up with their peers in this area. That begins, of course, at the center of the social circle as a child bonds with his parents. First, in the womb and then at birth, is the mother-baby touch connection. It is not uncommon for a child to start out closer to one parent and then, in time, open up to the other. As an example, we take this father's sweet report: "When my daughter was born, she looked in my eyes and saw my soul. She has owned me ever since." This is the essential human connection – life-affirming, life-sustaining and lifelong.

The social circle expands, generally in a stepwise way, next with older and then with younger siblings. A mother had this to say about her young son finally recognizing his baby sister:

My son never really noticed his baby sister. He would even crawl right over her like she wasn't even there. Then I noticed that he started watching her play and now he sits down next to her to play.

Mother of a 5-year-old

With time, a child's circle naturally opens to include grandparents and other familiar extended family members. From there, it widens out to his entire world as he opens to relationships with children his own age, and then he is finally ready for school. This widening circle all begins with the bonding and attachment that comes with normalized and affectionate touch.

However, those normal developmental steps can be disrupted when touch and sensory difficulties tip the nervous system toward survival mode, leaving a child anxious and unavailable to the social connection they desperately need. For babies and children with hyper-sensitive sensory nervous systems, even seemingly simple eye contact can be hyperactivating and overly stimulating. Instead of deepening the connection, it can make that connection uncomfortable and to be avoided, disrupting the natural cycle of social connection, even for years to come.

To help you repair this disruption, we've included the optional *Up-Up-Up Movement for Social Connection*. It was created specifically to integrate the neural messages from the skin to the brain that open the pathways for attention, communication and engaged social connection. *Up-Up-Up* should be included in the daily routine after Movement 1 and before Movement 2 of the *QST Sensory Protocol* (see Chapter 8 for full step-by-step instructions). As you help your child's ability to find the regulated relax-and-relate mode, you open the developmental pathway for him to begin to comfortably and quite naturally connect with other people more easily. The first step toward all forms of later social connection begins with you!

Warmest wishes,

Linda and Louisa

Week 47

Sensory Problems and Success in School

Dear parents,

Why do schools pay so much attention to whether hearing and vision tests are normal? They do it because they know that even mild hearing or vision impairment affects children's ability to learn, and that more severe impairment will cause a child to fall significantly behind. Educators know that sensory impairment is an important problem that must be taken care of if a child is to have the best chance of success in school. But what about the most fundamental of the senses, touch?

Touch is called the 'mother of all senses' because the neurons that wire for touch are among the first to develop in the embryo and serve as the matrix and foundation for the development of all other senses. And it is on that basis that a child's full range of skills and capacities develops. Because it underlies the other senses in this way, touch can compensate for problems with those other senses. For example, deaf and blind children can develop their sense of touch to compensate for their sensory loss. But it's harder for the other senses, hearing and vision, to compensate for touch. And when touch is abnormal, those higher senses are impacted as well. Noises seem too loud, lights seem too bright, and normal tastes and smells seem too strong. Without the organizing influence of touch, sensory information becomes disorganized and confusing, and a child is easily overwhelmed, leading to problems in school.

Unfortunately, our culture has forgotten the importance of touch over the last decades. But current neuroscience is bringing a new understanding to this area, highlighting its critical importance for a child's healthy development and how touch and related sensory problems are just as likely to result in a lack of progress in school as hearing and vision impairment, probably more so. Part of the reason that schools don't show the same amount of attention to this area is that they don't realize how touch affects the other sensory, emotional and learning problems. And they don't know that these problems can be effectively treated.

Most school administrators and parents know that hearing aids and glasses work for their respective senses but are mostly unaware of the touch-based interventions that address this most fundamental of senses. When touch problems are treated, the nervous system calms down and the other senses normalize right along with it. Research shows that touch-related sensory problems are treatable, and when they are treated, not only do the other sensory problems improve but difficult behaviors also diminish and children do better all around, bringing greater success at school.

All our best,

Linda and Louisa

Week 48

Unlocking My Child's Potential

A Parent's Story of Her Child With Crohn's Disease

Note from Linda and Louisa: Even though Andrew's diagnosis includes autism, we've included this letter because the issues and dilemmas that he struggled with perfectly mirror the challenges for all parents when faced with children's difficulties with sleep, GI and digestive problems and prolonged tantrums.

Dear fellow parents,

What do you most deeply want for your kids? For me, it is that they are healthy and reaching their greatest potential. For my child, that vision became much reduced. You go from dreaming of them taking the world head-on to just praying you can get them functional enough to manage. I have spent countless hours trying to unlock the potential I could see stuck inside my son. Qigong unlocked his potential, allowing him to access his own brain and for the first time to understand himself and how to connect with others. This is more than just another time commitment for parents; it's a life-altering tool. I am so blessed to have found it.

When Andrew was six months old, he started waking up screaming in the night and nothing seemed to comfort him. There were other challenges as he grew – we suspected lactose intolerance, he would panic if I was out of his sight for even a second and the only word he spoke by the age of three was "mama". His tantrums were terrible and could last for hours. He would complain that his head hurt and scream until he vomited or passed out. He had severe seasonal allergies and bad diarrhea, sometimes with bleeding. His doctor finally diagnosed Crohn's disease, and I was shocked to learn that it is not curable and can only be managed with lots of medicine and even surgery if the drugs fail to keep it in remission.

Around this time, a client of my husband connected me to an online QST support group for families with children with special needs, including autism. Soon after we started, Andrew threw up a whole bunch of phlegm. I was worried that I had done something wrong! But Dr. Silva reassured me that when children detox, it either goes up and out or down and out. Right afterwards, his little bloated belly got flat. He did a little more purging for about three months. Then he regressed, but we were prepared for that. The good news is that it only lasted a week, and we made it through.

After that, Andrew started healing and gaining weight. His cheeks got rosy, he started learning new things and he's had his first growth spurt in years. He's started approaching and talking with other people on his own. He started saying rhyming words for the first time and actually sang a song out loud! I was amazed at the transformation! He seems to have a new awareness of who he is and where he fits in this big bright world. And recently his lab results have been encouraging.

One day, about four months into the QST, Andrew was struggling to get a fitted sheet on his mattress. I'd shown him many times how to do it, and I couldn't stop and help him because I was busy getting the other kids to bed, so I left him to figure it out on his own. Normally this would have ended in an epic meltdown, but instead he was able to calm himself down and to actually tell me, "I don't feel special, important to you, because you won't help me". I was so touched. He had never been able to articulate how he felt like that before. I had to choke back tears as I put the boys on hold and went to help him. He really didn't need much help at all, and he was beaming and I was so proud of him! He hugged me so hard I couldn't breathe!

His Crohn's is doing very well now. We keep him on a diet, and he isn't sick with it anymore. He is growing like a weed! Overall, he is a much different boy than when we started this journey. This is more than a 15–30-minute commitment, it's the opportunity to breathe life into your child, an opportunity you are not likely to find elsewhere. I hope you find the person waiting to be unlocked inside your child, too!

A mom

Week 49

QST for the Home Medicine Cabinet

A Mother's Story

Dear fellow parents,

I found the Qigong routine invaluable! I first used a short version of Qigong when my youngest was just a 2-month-old. He was having problems latching during breastfeeding, causing me a lot of pain and him a lot of frustration. It completely amazed me that doing some specific Qigong movements could help with latching issues. But it did!

Later, when my youngest was three years old, he started having massive tantrums that often lasted three hours. It was miserable for the whole family! I happened to be learning QST for my work at that time, so I decided to try it on my son to see what would happen. After a few weeks, the frequency and length of his tantrums decreased dramatically. After a while, he very rarely had a tantrum. So, we started slacking and not doing the daily routine, then the tantrums came back! Once we resumed, the tantrums went away again. This happened several times. So I'm certain that the QST made the difference!

Because I saw how much it helped, I ended up giving the daily routine to both of my sons at bedtime for a few years. For my older son, it was useful in helping him slowdown from the day and get ready to sleep. His brain works very fast and hard, so getting him to unwind was challenging at times, but QST settled him right down. Several years later, my boys occasionally still request that I give them Qigong at bedtime. I think they can feel when their bodies need it. QST was so helpful, even for my typically-developing kiddos!

Mom of now 9-year-old and 12-year-old sons

Week 50

The Importance of Early Self-Regulation for Adulthood

Reflections From a QST Master Trainer

Dear parents,

The foundation for healthy self-regulation and social engagement in adulthood starts from a very early age, when primary attachment styles with caregivers are developed. Infants are dependent on caregivers to provide active soothing and comfort, which promotes a sense of safety and belonging within the relational bond. It is through such ongoing, attuned, co-regulating interaction that the infant's neurophysiological 'platform' is consolidated and strengthened – a requirement for achieving healthy regulation and the capacity for social engagement throughout life. As an example, Stephen Porges, in his polyvagal theory, points out that the muscles of the face when used for suckling are 'wired' to regulate the heart rate. In this way, suckling activity and skin-to-skin contact actually calm the infant down. In much the same way, we help to regulate each other as adults when we seek hugs and the sharing of meals with friends as ways of building and reinforcing that same soothing co-regulation through social connections.

A child's co-regulation and interdependency with a primary caregiver is fundamental to the development of a regulated nervous system. QST research shows that Qigong is a powerful tool for parents to reduce a child's sensory issues and promote self-regulation. The touch of a parent, attuned to their child's body responses, promotes the child's sense of safety and builds the self-regulation milestones that are typically achieved in the first year of life – the ability to self-soothe and to regulate orientation/attention, digestion and sleep/wake cycles. By the third year, the ability to regulate emotions and behavior in response to social cues is usually developed.

Once the nervous system becomes capable of self-regulation, the individual can identify sensations, regulate emotions and manage behavior. Imagine your child experiencing excitement or frustration when dealing with conflicts in relationships without withdrawing, handling stress without dissociating from his body or emotions and feeling a sense of safety in his body while enjoying life. With these skills in hand, he will be capable of taking in and processing information, being successful in school, developing a career, achieving autonomy and establishing satisfying intimate and social relationships. All these capacities are built on those first-year milestones and on early language development. Our goal is to help your child grow into an adult capable of spontaneous and regulated expression and mature autonomy.

Warmly,

Rosimery Bergeron, QST Master Trainer

www.QSTI.org/master-trainers/

Year's End – Weeks 51–52

Week 51

Year-End Evaluation

Dear parent,

Congratulations! You've just completed your first year of QST. You stuck to it, and you should feel very proud of yourself. It was tough at the beginning, but you persevered and now you get to see just how much progress your child has made over the past year. You'll recall that you completed two simple checklists at the beginning of the year – the *Sense and Self-Regulation Checklist* and the *Parenting Stress Index*. Then you completed them again halfway through the year to see how your child had progressed. You might remember that the *Sense and Self-Regulation Checklist* measured how severe your child's touch/pain and regulation problems were, and the *Parenting Stress Index* evaluated how challenging it was to parent your child. Now, you will complete these checklists a third time to see how the scores continued to change during the second half of the year.

Instructions to complete year-end checklists:

Start by completing both of the **Year-End Evaluation** checklists found at the end of this letter on pages 199–201). Don't look back at your previous scores so that you come to the checklists fresh. [You can also download and print out a copy of the forms – See link in Appendix H – to include as part of your child's medical, intervention or school records.]

Next, enter your final scores in the lines below marked **Year-End Eval** for both the *Sense and Self-Regulation Checklist* and the *Parent Stress Index*.

Sense and Self-Regulation Checklist

Start Date Total Score: _____
Mid-Year Check Total Score: _____
Year-End Eval Total Score: _____

DOI: 10.4324/9781003360421-24

Parent Stress Index

   Start Date Total Score: _____
Mid-Year Check Total Score: _____
   Year-End Eval Total Score: _____

Now, let's compare today's scores with the scores from the **Start Date** and with the **Mid-Year Check** by looking back to *Week 27 – Mid-Year Check-In* (page 162) to find your previous scores and then fill in those blanks (Start Date and Mid-Year) above.

What did you find? Did the scores continue to go down in the last half of the year? Depending on how severe your child's sensory, self-regulation and behavioral difficulties had been to begin with, the current scores may have come down a lot or a little. And this probably matches the improvements you are seeing in your child. Some of you may want to look a little deeper into the *Sense and Self-Regulation* scores in particular. For that, you can look at specific questions or behavioral symptoms that you checked across each of the three periods (beginning, six months and today). Have any initial sensory problems improved more than others? Have any stayed the same or worsened?

Look also at the *Parent Stress Index* to measure any specific items or areas that highlight your own progress. While many of you will already intuit or sense these changes, we've found that it can be very helpful to see changes over time measured in black and white. Some of these improvements may be ones you've taken for granted. But take a closer look, you may be surprised at how much your own stress levels have come down or how your concerns have changed!

Instructions to complete the year-end *QST Progress Chart*

Just as you did at the beginning and at mid-year, fill in the *QST Progress Chart* below, circling the number in each column that best reflects your child's current capacities and difficulties. Connect the scores with a line and don't forget to add any items you may have previously written in the two extra lines at the far-right side.

QST Progress Chart - Mid-Year Check

Sleep	Digestion Elimination	Focus Attention	Self Regulation	Social Connection	Tantrums Aggression	Touch Sensitivity	/	/
10	10	10	10	10	10	10	10	10
9	9	9	9	9	9	9	9	9
8	8	8	8	8	8	8	8	8
7	7	7	7	7	7	7	7	7
6	6	6	6	6	6	6	6	6
5	5	5	5	5	5	5	5	5
4	4	4	4	4	4	4	4	4
3	3	3	3	3	3	3	3	3
2	2	2	2	2	2	2	2	2
1	1	1	1	1	1	1	1	1

Self-Regulation Milestones

Figure 20.2 **QST Progress Chart – Year-End Evaluation** – circle the number in each column that reflects your child child's current capabilities. A score of '10' is very positive/no difficulty, and '1' is most difficult. Then, connect the circles to complete the sensory and self-regulation 'picture'. Be sure to copy in your Start Date and Mid-Year Check lines for comparison.

QST Progress Chart
Year-End Evaluation

Now that you've created a line connecting your year-end evaluation scores, you can compare your progress over the last year. Look back to find your previously completed mid-year *QST Progress Chart* in Weekly Letter 27 (page 164), that includes both your start date and mid-year graph lines. Copy in the numbers and connecting lines onto this chart using different colored pencils. The three separate lines on this new chart – 'start date', 'mid-year check' and 'year-end eval' – allow you to easily compare your child's progress throughout the year. Pay special attention to how much or how little improvement there has been in each area. Has more improvement or change happened in the first half-year or in the second? What areas changed the most? The least? Hopefully, this will confirm what you have been observing so you can celebrate your successes and help focus on areas that may be in need of more attention.

These checklists and charts give you a clearer picture of how and where both you and your child have changed, but the area that almost certainly has improved is that of your child's problems with touch. Even though there may still be some sensitivity in some areas, touch is becoming more normal. You're able to use parent touch a lot more now, and that is super important to your child's learning, development and ability to connect with other people and the world around him. And you are probably less stressed and more relaxed as a parent now than you were at the beginning, and maybe even more than you were six months ago. So, it's time to celebrate! Sit back and enjoy hearing from a few parents who have traveled this journey before you.

It's as if something has finally connected with her mind and body. Today I was moved to tears watching her play on the playground. She is so much more coordinated and she doesn't have to fight her body anymore. She's in sync.

Mother of a 5-year-old

Eric is actually asking for QST after his bath, he calls it "medicine". He is now so accustomed to expecting it right after his bath that he has actually been helping us stay on track each night. We are really finding QST to not only be a huge benefit to Eric but to ourselves. After long working days, we look forward to going through the steps to help us take a deep breath and relax!

Mother of a 5-year-old

Congratulations on your accomplishments!
Next week, we will share our final thoughts and appreciations.
All our best
Louisa and Linda

Sense and Self-Regulation Checklist

Name of child: _____   Year-End Check Date: _____

Please circle the response for each item that most accurately describes your child.

1. TACTILE = ORAL & TACTILE	Often	Sometimes	Rarely	Never
• Does not cry tears when hurt	3	2	1	0
• Doesn't notice if the diaper is wet or dirty	3	2	1	0
• Face washing is difficult	3	2	1	0
• Haircuts are difficult	3	2	1	0
• Refuses to wear a hat	3	2	1	0
• Prefers to wear a hat	3	2	1	0
• Cutting fingernails is difficult	3	2	1	0
• Prefers to wear one or two gloves	3	2	1	0
• Avoids wearing gloves	3	2	1	0
• Cutting toenails is difficult	3	2	1	0
• Will only wear certain footwear (e.g. loose shoes, no socks)	3	2	1	0
• Prefers to wear the same clothes day after day	3	2	1	0
• Will only wear certain clothes (e.g. no elastic, not tight, no tags, long or short sleeves)	3	2	1	0
• Cries tears when falls, scrapes skin, or gets hurt (Scale is reversed on purpose)	0	1	2	3
• Head bangs on a hard surface	3	2	1	0
• Head bangs on a soft surface	3	2	1	0
• Avoids foods with certain textures	3	2	1	0
• Tooth brushing is difficult	3	2	1	0
• Mouths or chews objects	3	2	1	0
Self-regulation – Orientation/Attention/Self-soothing/Sleep	Often	Sometimes	Rarely	Never
• Has to be prompted to make eye contact when spoken to	3	2	1	0
• Seems not to notice when spoken to in a normal voice	3	2	1	0
• Does not respond to his/her name	3	2	1	0
• Does not notice or react when tapped on the back	3	2	1	0
• Does not roll over onto the back when asked	3	2	1	0
• Stares off into space	3	2	1	0
• Seems unaware when others are hurt	3	2	1	0
• Has difficulty calming him/herself when upset	3	2	1	0
• Gets upset or tantrums when asked to make a transition	3	2	1	0
• Has difficulty falling asleep at bedtime	3	2	1	0
• Has difficulty falling back asleep when awakens during the night	3	2	1	0
• Awakens very early and stays awake	3	2	1	0
• Has difficulty awakening in morning	3	2	1	0
• Makes little jokes (*Answer only if your child has language.*) (Scale is reversed on purpose)	0	1	2	3
SubTotal-pg 1: _____ [Sum of all columns]	☐	☐	☐	☐

Please circle the response for each item that most accurately describes your child.

2. SENSORY = VISION	Often	Sometimes	Rarely	Never
• Looks at objects out of sides of eyes	3	2	1	0
• Is bothered by certain lights	3	2	1	0
Self-regulation – Behavior: Irritability, Aggression, Self-injurious	Often	Sometimes	Rarely	Never
• Tantrums or meltdowns	3	2	1	0
(Tantrums last_____minutes, and occur_____times/day)				
• Cries easily when frustrated	3	2	1	0
• Hits or kicks others	3	2	1	0
• Scratches or pulls other's hair	3	2	1	0
• Bites others	3	2	1	0
• Throws things at others	3	2	1	0
• Pulls own hair (Where on the head?)	3	2	1	0
• Bites self (Which part of the body e.g. left thumb?)	3	2	1	0
• Hits self (Which part of the body?)_____	3	2	1	0
• Gets aggressive or 'hyper' with exposure to certain smells	3	2	1	0
3. SENSORY = HEARING	Often	Sometimes	Rarely	Never
• Reacts poorly to certain everyday noises	3	2	1	0
• Covers ears with certain sounds	3	2	1	0
• Reacts strongly when others cry loudly or scream	3	2	1	0
• Is startled by sudden noises	3	2	1	0
Self-regulation – Toilet training	Often	Sometimes	Rarely	Never
• Is dry at night (scale is reversed on purpose)	0	1	2	3
• Diaper is wet in the morning	3	2	1	0
• Wears a diaper during the day	3	2	1	0
• Is toilet trained (scale is reversed on purpose)	0	1	2	3
4. SENSORY = SMELL	Often	Sometimes	Rarely	Never
• Gags with certain smells	3	2	1	0
Self-regulation – Digestion	Often	Sometimes	Rarely	Never
• Will only eat familiar foods	3	2	1	0
• Does not seem to be interested in food	3	2	1	0
• Eats very few foods (five to ten items)	3	2	1	0
• Bowels are loose	3	2	1	0
• Bowel movements ("poops") are frequent (more than 3 per day)	3	2	1	0
• Requires regular use of laxative to avoid constipation	3	2	1	0
• Bowel movement ("poop") is hard and dry	3	2	1	0
• Has a bowel movement every other day	3	2	1	0
• Has a bowel movement twice a week	3	2	1	0
• Has a bowel movement once a week	3	2	1	0
• Bowel movements are often green	3	2	1	0
	☐	☐	☐	☐

SubTotal pg 1: _____   **SubTotal pg 2:** _____   **Total**_____

Parent Stress Index

Name of child: _____   **Year-End Eval Date:** _____

Please rate the following aspects of your child's <u>health according to how much stress it causes you and/or your family</u> by placing an X in the box that best describes your situation.	Stress Ratings				
	Not stressful	Sometimes creates stress	Often creates stress	Very stressful on a daily basis	So stressful sometimes we feel we can't cope
Your child's social development	0	1	2	3	5
Your child's ability to communicate	0	1	2	3	5
Tantrums/meltdowns	0	1	2	3	5
Aggressive behavior (siblings, peers)	0	1	2	3	5
Self-injurious behavior	0	1	2	3	5
Difficulty making transitions from one activity to another	0	1	2	3	5
Sleep problems	0	1	2	3	5
Your child's diet	0	1	2	3	5
Bowel problems (diarrhea, constipation)	0	1	2	3	5
Potty training	0	1	2	3	5
Not feeling close to your child	0	1	2	3	5
Concern for the future of your child being accepted by others	0	1	2	3	5
Concern for the future of your child living independently	0	1	2	3	5
Subtotal					
Total					

Week 52

Final Thoughts and Appreciations

Dear parents,

We know that parenting children with sensory and behavioral problems requires a lot of extras – extra patience, extra courage, extra energy, extra stamina, extra hope and extra support. We trust that this year of QST has provided you with the extra support you needed to help address and even resolve many of the issues that brought you to QST.

And now that you've come to the end of the year, we hope that QST has become a special time for you and your child and a natural part of what you do together as a family. We trust that his behavior has improved and that he is more connected to his body and the people and world around him. That he is sleeping, eating and communicating better. And that he is growing and developing on a healthier track. We trust you can hardly remember what those long tantrums looked like – well, okay, even typically-developing children occasionally melt down. But things are going much more smoothly, and you are more relaxed as a parent. You are able to use your touch more freely and effectively with your child and you know how important that is to his learning and development.

So, we encourage you to continue your QST. If you keep doing the daily routine, will it continue to help your child? Yes it will! Our research shows that improvements seen in the first year continue to grow in the second year. And parents often ask, do you have to continue to give QST every day forever? Well, no, not necessarily. But we encourage you to continue to use it with your child for as long as you feel it is supporting him and he is enjoying it. The daily routine helps your child navigate the normal rhythms, changes and challenges of life and prevent stresses from piling up in his body and nervous system. If you feel he is doing so well that you decide to stop, remember you can always come back during challenging times and pick up right where you left off. There will always be times when your child needs your extra help to get through the day.

You also have a lot to offer other parents who are just starting this journey. You can share your experiences with others on our QST Parent Support Facebook page (www.facebook.com/QigongSTI). And when you need extra support yourself, you can post your own questions there as well.

We feel like we have traveled this road together with you as you started this adventure, struggled through the initial weeks and gained skill and confidence. We have shared your joys as your child finally slept through the night, started using the potty, sat quietly for a haircut and even began trying new foods! We celebrated when meltdowns faded away and you started receiving positive reports from teachers at school. We have shared your challenges and delight in your successes. We are so happy to have shared Qigong Sensory Treatment with you and your child. We wish you all the best as you continue to grow as a family.

With our very warmest wishes,

Linda and Louisa

Appendix A

QST Sensory Movement Chart and Guiding Tips

QST Sensory Movement Chart on next page.

[Also see Appendix H, page 221, for link to download printable copy.]

What the 12 Movements Do

1. **Making a connection** [down the arms] makes a gentle relaxing connection between you and your child that begins the QST time together. It opens up circulation to the arms and hands and engages the relaxation response preparing your child for the rest of the movements.
2. **Relax chest** relaxes emotional and physical tension and triggers your child's ability to self-soothe. They may yawn or rub their eyes.
3. **Belly circles** regulates digestion and appetite and increases your child's tolerance for stress and change.
4. **Down the legs** helps clear toxicity from the belly and strengthen the legs.
5. **Down the back – one hand** opens circulation to the skin and the back and helps your child's body settle down. Increases body awareness, helps with potty training and helps stop toe walking.
6. **Down the back – two hands** helps your child's body settle down. Helps stop toe walking. Helps with potty training.
7. **Down the sides** clears out the effects of repeated ear infections, calms irritability.
8. **Ear to hand** relaxes the neck, clears the ears.
9. **Fingers** helps the fingers become more comfortable to touch, stimulates connection to speech areas of brain.
10. **Relax legs** relaxes muscle tension, helps your child calm down, brings energy and circulation down to the feet.
11. **Toes** helps the toes become comfortable to touch, brings fuller circulation to the legs and feet.
12. **Nourish and integrate** sends nourishing, integrating energy up, from the feet to the brain, in a rhythmic wave-like motion, to fill your child's inner energy reserves.

QST Sensory Movement Chart

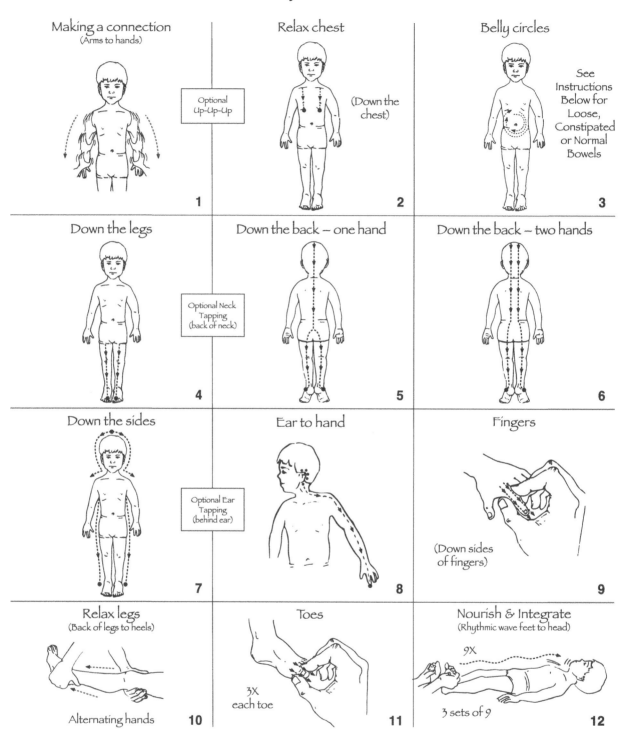

Making a connection
(Arms to hands)

Optional Up-Up-Up

1

Relax chest

(Down the chest)

2

Belly circles

See Instructions Below for Loose, Constipated or Normal Bowels

3

Down the legs

Optional Neck Tapping (back of neck)

4

Down the back – one hand

5

Down the back – two hands

6

Down the sides

Optional Ear Tapping (behind ear)

7

Ear to hand

8

Fingers

(Down sides of fingers)

9

Relax legs
(Back of legs to heels)

Alternating hands   **10**

Toes

3X each toe

11

Nourish & Integrate
(Rhythmic wave feet to head)

9X

3 sets of 9   **12**

What if my child has normal, loose or constipated bowels?

Option 1: If your child has **loose or normal** bowels, do belly circles starting clockwise: rub 9x clockwise, followed by 9x counterclockwise and then 9x clockwise.

Option 2: If your child has **constipation** start counterclockwise: rub 9x counterclockwise, followed by 9x clockwise and 9x counterclockwise. When the bowels return to normal, change back to option 1.

©LMTSilva 2011

Your child's belly is 'the clock"

9x   9x   9x

9x   9x   9x

Important Signs of Progress

Look for Changes In

Stools. Soon after starting QST, your child may pass one or several dark green or black stools, indicating that the digestive system is clearing out. This is a good sign of progress. If you child has:

- **Diarrhea:** loose stools will become more formed and less frequent.
- **Constipation:** stools will become more frequent and softer.

Sleep. Children fall asleep more easily at bedtime and stay asleep all night, especially if QST is part of the bedtime routine.

Behavior. After children visibly calm with the 'relax chest' movement, they become calmer at other times and develop more of a window of tolerance for frustration and change. Tantrums diminish or disappear.

Sensory. Children become more and more receptive to parents' caring touch. Haircuts and loud noises are easier to tolerate, and children are able to wear a wider selection of clothes.

Social skills. Your child's social circle will widen, and she will be more comfortable with less familiar family members, other adults and children at school.

Language. Listening and self-expression improve.

Appetite. Children eat more and are willing to try new things. (Avoid processed foods and foods with red dye.)

Appendix B

Troubleshooting Guide

If you are struggling with a particular movement or feel you aren't getting the results you want, you may be missing an important concept such as incorrectly tapping around the ears, not patting the proper spot on the top of the head or not adjusting the speed or weight of your hand. The simple checklist below highlights the important items to pay special attention to. These are the little details that can make a huge difference and ensure that you are doing the movements most effectively. Keep this list handy and refer to it when you encounter problems. If you are fortunate enough to have a partner or support group member observing you, they can keep an eye on these items for you, especially during the first weeks when you have a lot of new things to remember and attend to. Also review the online video instructions at [see link in Appendix H, page 221].

Important Items to Watch for

Movement 1 – Making a Connection – Arms to Hands

Am I . . .

- finding my own sense of calm and relaxation before I begin?
- making a steady, reassuring connection with my child?
- using slow, deep pressure movements (rhythm of resting heartbeat, 60 beats/min)?
- starting at the shoulders, then moving down her arms to the hands?
- watching for eye contact and smile, relaxation of shoulders, arms, hands?

Movement 2 – Relax Chest

Am I . . .

- using movements that are slow and rhythmic, not rushed?
- pressing gently but firmly, so as to move her ribs slightly (as much as would happen with a breath)?
- starting at the collarbone and moving down to the bottom of her rib cage?
- watching for key cues (yawning, rubbing eyes, humming or hands moving to rest on top of mine) and staying at that point until her response stops? Then continuing on to finish the movements?

Movement 3 – Belly Circles

Am I . . .

- considering whether my child has constipation, diarrhea or normal stools and then doing the movement in the correct direction (see *QST Sensory Movement Chart*)?
- making circles around the belly button?
- adjusting my speed and pressure according to my child's cues?
- watching for responses such as humming (stay on the spot until humming stops) or legs drawing up (pat or press down legs), then resuming the movement?

Movement 4 – Down the Legs

Am I . . .

- following the center line down the top of the thigh, shin and top of the foot?
- adjusting the weight of my hand for ticklishness or other responses (deep pressure for ticklishness)?
- patting down the legs if they draw up, and then resuming the movement?

Movement 5 – Down the Back – One Hand

Am I . . .

- checking that there are no hair clasps, ties, etc. on the head?
- patting specifically on the soft spot (center of head), not just anywhere on the head?
- doing an adequate number of pats before moving on?
- following the correct line down the center of the head and spine, down the middle of the back and legs to the outside of the heels?
- continuing the movement all the way to the outside of the heels?
- giving extra pats in those areas where her responses indicate the need (e.g., humming, discomfort or tight areas)?
- adjusting the weight of my hand appropriately?

Movement 6 – Down the Back – Two Hands

Am I . . .

- beginning with both hands patting on either side of the soft spot on the top of the head?
- following the correct lines down both sides of my child's spine?
- giving extra pats in areas where her responses indicate the need (e.g., humming, discomfort or tight areas)?

Movement 7 – Down the Sides

Am I . . .

- beginning with tapping at the soft spot, center, on the top of my child's head?
- being sure to tap with the flats of my fingers (avoiding using my fingernails)?

- lingering and tapping several times once I reach the area at the back of the ears?
- keeping my fingers slightly spread and adjusting the weight of my tapping according to my child's responses?
- patting well with flats of fingers onto the sides of the neck?
- following the correct path down the sides of the body to the outside of the ankles?

Movement 8 – Ear to Hand

Am I . . .

- using the proper hand position (relaxed cupped hand, open fingers, flats of fingertips at the back of the ear) and adjusting the weight of my tapping in response to my child's cues?
- giving each ear ample pats before moving on?
- focusing on particular discomfort around the ears by having a partner (if available) tap on the top of the shoulder at the same time I'm tapping around the ear?
- following the correct line from the ear to the side of the neck, across the top of the shoulder, down the upper arm to the elbow, across the top of the forearm and ending on the top of the hand and fingers?
- doing extra repetitions if the ear is blocked (patting or pressing, according to my child's comfort level)?
- aware when I need to switch to pressing (when patting is too uncomfortable)?

Movement 9 – Fingers – Down Sides of Fingers

Am I . . .

- using the appropriate technique, either rubbing or pressing, in response to my child's responses?
- watching for responses and spending extra time on certain fingers if needed?

Movement 10 – Relax Legs – Back of Legs to Heels

Am I . . .

- using a firm, supportive grip on the heel with one hand as the other hand starts the movement just above the backside of the knee?
- using movements that are smooth and continuous?
- continuing the movement until her leg is relaxed and the calf muscle loose?
- switching to a gentle pressing motion down the calf if I encounter ticklishness or discomfort?

Movement 11 – Toes

Am I . . .

- using rubbing or pressing according to my child's responses and receptivity?
- adjusting to a bicycling motion if necessary to make movement comfortable?
- spending extra time on individual toes (if needed)?

Movement 12 – Nourish and Integrate – Rhythmic Wave Feet to Head

Am I . . .

- checking that my child's body is aligned and the neck is in neutral position (head and neck in a straight line, centered)?
- positioning my hands correctly on her feet?
- watching for a slight chin rocking during the movement?
- counting slowly and quietly aloud to match the rocking movements?
- asking if my child wants another set when done?

And Finally

At the end of the routine, your child may enjoy a quiet hug. You can offer encouragement and affection, and then let her rest so she can integrate the effects of the treatment. Watch quietly until she chooses to get up or fall asleep.

Appendix C

Contraindications to the QST Sensory Protocol

There are five contraindications to starting the QST Sensory Protocol with your child. We list them here, along with the reasons:

1. **Uncontrolled seizures despite being on seizure medicine.** We do not recommend QST for children with uncontrolled seizures even if they are on medication for the condition. Gentle tapping on the head can precipitate a seizure and even children with controlled seizures can be at greater risk. Advanced training is required for QST Master Trainers and Certified Therapists to work with children with this diagnosis. Contact QSTI (www.qsti.org/contact/) to be referred to a QST professional who is qualified to support parents of children with seizure disorder.
2. **Other conditions such as autism or Down syndrome.** The QST Sensory Protocol is specific for children with sensory or behavioral problems. For children on the autism spectrum, we recommend the QST Autism Protocol. For children with Down syndrome, please refer to our QST Down Syndrome Protocol. See our bookstore (www.qsti.org/shop/) for the books that provide parent instructions and online instructional videos for the QST protocols tailored to each condition.
3. **Parents lack sensitivity in their hands.** Parents must be able to see and feel their child's avoidance of touch so that they can attune the QST touch technique to their child's specific sensory issues. If parents are unable to do so, QST can be unpleasant and ineffective.
4. **Children are beginning other forms of intensive treatment at the same time as QST.** Starting QST at the same time as other intensive treatments can overload your child's nervous system. If your child has a strong reaction, you will not know which treatment is causing it, or how to manage it. We recommend starting only one intensive treatment at a time. When your child has adjusted to one treatment, the second treatment can be added.
5. **Children are taking strong medication.** The success of QST comes when the parent can read and respond to the child's cues during the routine. Because the intervention works via the sensory nervous system, certain sedatives (e.g., gabapentin) interfere with the sensory signals that the QST protocols rely on. For these children, progress can be slower. Similarly, if a child is going through medication changes, the medication can affect the child's body, making it difficult to know whether the child is reacting to the QST or to the medication. Some strong medications like Tegretol (carbamazepine) or Risperdal (risperidone) tend to block the effect of QST altogether. In general, it is better to wait until the child is stabilized on the medication before beginning the home program.

Appendix D

Getting Personalized QST Help

We know that most people will have good results if they follow the directions in this book and rely on the online instructional videos and the year of 52 Weekly Letters (in Part III – Guiding Your Way). But for families who feel they need additional one-on-one support and guidance, certified QST professionals are there to help. They will work individually with you and your child on a weekly basis to coach and support you through any challenges and help you improve your technique. Our research clearly shows that the more training and support a parent receives from a QST-trained professional, the better the results for their child.

Certified QST Trainer. A certified QST professional has graduated from an approved course of training that includes six months of clinical supervision. They are trained to both teach the QST protocols to parents and to work hands-on, directly with children. They will meet with you and your family in-person (and many offer online virtual sessions) to teach you the 12-step QST routine and to show you how to refine your technique and attune it specifically to your child's individual sensory needs. They will also work directly with your child. Hands-on work with a certified therapist helps in two ways. First, the trainer can demonstrate how to work through more challenging and sensitive areas. Secondly, because of their training and experience, QST Certified Trainer can identify and open up sensitive or resistant areas that parents may be reluctant to deal with. The combination can make your home treatment easier and more effective, improve your technique and encourage you to keep moving forward so you can optimize your treatment at home to get the very best results. This extra level of parent training and support resulted in a large decrease in autism severity in our research studies. Cost per session varies. To find a certified therapist in your area go to the QSTI website (www.qsti.org/finding-a-qst-therapist/). If you live in an area without access to a local QST professional, many of our certified therapists and Master Trainers offer virtual sessions via Zoom, Skype or another preferred online platform.

Online QST parent training with online supervision. We offer online training and help for families where in-person training is not available or where parents prefer online support. Our 12-week course, taught by a certified QST Therapist, teaches parents how to do the daily routine, provides weekly reading and discussions and includes a series of regular, personalized online coaching sessions where the instructor observes your at-home treatment, demonstrates how to adapt the technique and works through any areas of difficulty. For information go to the QSTI website (www.qsti.org/online-training-course-for-parents/).

QST Facebook page. Our Facebook page provides a forum for a community of parents and caregivers to share stories, ask questions and get support from other parents and therapists (www. facebook.com/QigongSTI).

Creating a Local QST Parent Support Group

Many parents who need additional support will not have access to a local QST professional. So, we encourage you to create your own support community. That can begin right at home. If available, enlist other family members, another parent, grandparent or caregiver. In addition, we strongly recommend that you gather a group of local parents with children who face similar challenges. You probably already know other families with similar problems through your early intervention program or hopefully from local parent support groups. If a group of families doesn't come to mind immediately, ask your early intervention specialist. Also check online for any existing parent support groups. With others, you can learn the steps, share information, make new discoveries and provide useful feedback to hone your skills. Fellow parents can encourage you to stick with it through the sometimes difficult first weeks until you begin to see and recognize tangible results. Here are the support group steps to success:

- **Before you begin.** Every member should have a copy of this book and the *QST Sensory Movement Chart* [see Appendix A, page 204]. It also helps if everyone watches the online instructional videos [see link in Appendix H, page 221] and/or reads the book prior to coming, but it shouldn't be a requirement.
- **Record personal goals.** At the start of the first meeting, each parent or couple should turn to the "Setting Goals" (page 57) section in Chapter 7 – Getting Started and write down the three goals or specific areas of improvement that they would like to see (e.g., sleeps through the night, responds to her name, aggression subsides).
- **Watch the online instructional videos as a group.** The videos are a valuable tool that demonstrate step-by-step how to do the 12 QST movements [See link in Appendix H]. Try to arrange those initial meetings as gatherings for adults only so that you can pay close attention to the videos without distractions.
- **Mark your progress.** Before beginning the daily routine with your child, each parent should complete the **Start Date QST Progress Chart** (Chapter 7, page 59 and the Start Date **Sense and Self-Regulation Checklist** and **Parent Stress Index** at the end of Chapter 7 (pages 60–62), to establish a baseline record from which to mark both your child's progress and yours over the year.
- **Practice the 12 movements together.** After watching all 12 movements on the video to see the flow of it, watch the first two movements again. With your *QST Sensory Movement Chart* in hand [see Appendix A], break into groups of three or four to practice giving the first two

movements to one another. Then watch the next two movements, practice those and continue watching and practicing two at a time until you've completed all 12. It is best if everyone *gives* and *receives* the entire routine at least once because while it's important to both learn and practice each movement, it is also important to experience how it feels on your own body. For the sake of social comfort, you can adapt the routine for certain movements (for example, patting the air above the chest or buttocks). Using the *Troubleshooting Guide* [see Appendix B, page 206] as a guide, members should watch and give feedback.

- **After practicing the 12 movements.** Gather together after the practice to compare notes and ask questions that have come up. Trade contact information so you can talk over questions or observations that you may have over the next week.
- **Next meeting.** Meet again in a week, as a group or in pairs, to demonstrate the full routine for one another. Use the *Troubleshooting Guide* [Appendix B] and compare against the *QST Sensory Movement Chart* to be sure that you are doing each step correctly.
- **Subsequent meetings.** We recommend that you arrange future meetings for once or twice a month. They are a great place to share questions, experiences and insights. Knowing that you will be meeting again and reporting your progress will motivate you to keep going when you are tempted to skip the daily routine. However, it's important to develop specific goals for your group. For example, one group may choose to only learn the daily routine and then stop after the first few weeks when everyone feels ready. Or, as we've seen happen in other groups, you may continue on as you find new friends who can share the journey with you and provide help and support in ways that far surpass the original purpose.
- **At home.** Everyone should plan to practice at home with a partner or a typically-developing child before beginning with their sensory child. Practicing the 12 movements on each other in the parent group and again at home with a family member will help you become familiar with how to do the movements so that once you start with your child, you can focus on adapting your touch to how your child responds. It may feel like a lot in the beginning, but you will find that over time, you won't need the book or the *QST Sensory Movement Chart*. All of your energy can then be focused on achieving a sense of calm and attuning to each movement.
- **Check-in** with an online virtual Q&A session with a QST Certified Trainer. Contact QSTI [www.QSTI.org/finding-a-qst-therapist/] for an online session.
- **As a final note.** While it can be helpful for parents who are seeing good results early to inspire others to continue, please keep in mind that every child will proceed in their own individual time. So don't measure your child's success against others in the group, even though it is natural and tempting to do so. Progress is measured from where your child begins, according to her own individual sensory picture and developmental timeline.

Appendix F

QST in Early Intervention

by Orit Tal-Atzili, OTD, OTR/L Certified QST Trainer and Master Trainer

Note: In this appendix, Dr. Tal-Atzili describes her experiences in designing and integrating QST treatment into a county-wide early intervention program in the state of Maryland. It is her hope, and ours, that her program will serve as a model for mainstreaming QST into early intervention programs across the country. It is an inspiring example of how QST can be offered as an affordable, evidence-based intervention to all families with children with sensory and self-regulation challenges. We encourage you to share this appendix with your own early intervention program.

I have provided occupational therapy (OT) services to children and their families for more than 25 years. Currently, I work at one of the largest early intervention programs in Maryland, which provides free services to approximately 5,000 families each year under Part C of the Individuals With Disabilities Education Act. Like many other early intervention programs, our program follows a family-centered approach and uses a routine-based coaching model to support families in their efforts to help their children with developmental delays to thrive.

Throughout my OT career, I was always both fascinated and baffled by how the sensory nervous system affects function and how challenging it can be for the entire family when sensory processing and self-regulation do not work as well as they should. I was continuously looking for strategies that could help regulate the sensory system, but did not find home interventions that consistently made a significant difference. And then, I found QST!

In 2014, I began my doctoral studies, which focused on evidence-based interventions for sensory challenges in children with autism. In an extensive literature search, I came across Dr. Silva's research with the QST Autism Protocol. I was impressed with the rigorous design and significant outcomes of the studies. They all demonstrated strong evidence of effectiveness for alleviating sensory and self-regulation challenges in children with autism. I felt like I won the lottery! This was exactly what I was looking for. I decided to focus my doctoral research on QST. My goal was to test if QST, when provided in our early intervention program, would yield the same dramatic results as those described in the published randomized controlled studies. After obtaining my certification as a QST Certified Trainer, I conducted a small pilot study with three families at my early intervention program. Two of the children had a diagnosis of autism, and the third child was a 'sensory child'. Over the five months of the pilot study, the parents implemented the QST Autism Protocol daily with their child and participated in 24 coaching home visits with me.

The results of my small pilot study exceeded my expectations! They were just like the amazing results of the large, published studies. All three children demonstrated a significant decrease in the frequency, intensity and duration of atypical behaviors related to sensory processing and self-regulation. The parents' stress levels also significantly decreased. Children demonstrated improvements in early self-regulation milestones for awareness, sleep, digestion and feeding as well as in higher-order functions such as social interactions, verbal and non-verbal communication, following directions, attention, problem-solving and purposeful play. Aggression and meltdowns decreased while eye contact and bonding with family members increased. Everything became easier, and children and families were able to access and engage in many more opportunities and life activities, in and outside of the home. The results of my pilot study were published in 2017 (Tal-Atzili & Salls 2017).

After I presented the strong research evidence supporting the effectiveness of QST, together with the promising outcomes of my pilot study and the high parent satisfaction ratings, the decision was made to expand QST into a county-wide program. My program funded training to certify additional QST Certified Trainers so that QST could be available to many more families in our county. Our county-wide QST program continues to be data-driven. We compare before and after scores on the *Sense and Self-Regulation Checklist* and on the *Parenting Stress Index*. At the end of the five-month coaching period, parents are also offered the opportunity to complete a survey and provide insights into their QST experiences. Our data to date (March 2021), gathered from families of diverse cultural and socio-economic backgrounds, continue to show the same amazing improvements. Data from 51 families who completed the post-testing by November 2020 (not all families complete the post-test) show normalization of sensory processing and self-regulation, including:

- 45% decrease in difficulties related to touch
- 46% decrease in sensory processing challenges
- 40% decrease in self-regulation problems
- 51% decrease in parenting stress
- Parent overall satisfaction rating of 4.9 out of 5

Currently (March 2021), with more than 100 families served, we have more demand for QST services than we can provide, and we hope to train additional QST Certified Trainers.

Since my pilot study, I have coached many more families (of children with or without autism) in QST. Through the QST research, as well as my own clinical observations and reports from co-workers, parents and caregivers, the evidence is clear: QST works! Every time! 100% of the children who participated in the QST program with me made progress. Many of the goals the families developed in their individualized family service plans (IFSP) were achieved at the end of the five-month QST coaching period. Most of the children made significant progress in all areas of development and in their ability to regulate themselves and participate in everyday life activities.

The evidence for the effectiveness of QST did not end there. Between 2018 and 2020, the American Journal of Occupational Therapy published three comprehensive systematic reviews (produced by the American Occupational Therapy Association's evidence-based project). Each of these systematic reviews supports the effectiveness of QST and recommends its use for sensory challenges, self-regulation, mental health and motor development in young children. (Kingsley et al. 2020, p. 9) (Tanner et al. 2020) (Bodison & Parham 2018, p. 5)

I became a QST Master Trainer in order to help certify more early interventionists as QST Certified Trainers so that many more families could have access to this effective, evidence-based intervention. I envision that through federal funding under the IDEA Part C early intervention law, early intervention programs throughout the country will offer free or affordable QST coaching for families with children with sensory challenges as part of their IFSP, as done in my county's program. I am excited for the possibility to share my experience and the model of my early intervention QST program with your program and interventionists to support this vision.

Orit Tal-Atzili, OTD, OTR/L
Certified QST Trainer and Master Trainer
Rockville, Maryland USA
www.qsti.org/meet-our-master-trainers.html
March 2021

References

Bodison, S.C., & Parham, L.D. (2018). Specific sensory techniques and sensory environmental modifications for children and youth with sensory integration difficulties: A systematic review. *American Journal of Occupational Therapy*, 72, 7201190040. [https://doi.org/10.5014/ajot.2018.029413]

Kingsley, K., Sagester, G., & Weaver, L.L. (2020). Interventions supporting mental health and positive behavior in children ages birth–5 yr: A systematic review. *American Journal of Occupational Therapy*, 74, 7402180050. [https://doi.org/10.5014/ajot.2020.039768]

Tal-Atzili, O., & Salls, J. (2017, May 19). Qigong Sensory Training pilot study: A tactile home program for children with or at-risk for autism. *Journal of Occupational Therapy, Schools, & Early Intervention*, 10(4), 366–388. [https://doi.org/10.1080/19411243.2017.1325819]

Tanner, K., Schmidt, E., Martin, K., & Bassi, M. (2020). Interventions within the scope of occupational therapy practice to improve motor performance for children ages 0–5 years: A systematic review. *American Journal of Occupational Therapy*, 74, 7402180060. [https://doi.org/10.5014/ajot.2020.039644]

Lessons Learned From QST Autism Research

As a physician and researcher, Louisa Silva dedicated her life to the study and resolution of sensory and self-regulation problems and how those abnormalities can disrupt a child's normal development. She published 21 university-based research studies evaluating the beneficial effects of QST for children with autism spectrum disorder and Down syndrome. Most importantly, her 16 years of studies demonstrated the direct relationship between sensory problems and the wide range of symptoms associated with autism. They showed a direct correlation between the severity of sensory difficulties and the severity of self-regulation problems.

Louisa next turned her investigations to children in other diagnostic groups with sensory and behavioral difficulties. She developed the QST Sensory Protocol focusing first on children with Down syndrome. Randomized controlled studies with both the original Autism Protocol and her new Sensory Protocol for Children with Down Syndrome showed consistent and compelling results. Her two small studies with Down syndrome showed a large improvement in expressive language and motor skills, just as her 16 years of autism studies have consistently shown significant improvements in sensory, self-regulation, behavioral and developmental problems.

The most recent and longer-term research study (Silva 2016) was funded by the U.S. Department of Health and Human Services – Maternal Child Health Bureau. That study, which included children ages 2 to 12, replicated and confirmed previous findings for children with autism and showed the long-term benefits of continuing QST for one and two years. Here are some of the more specific results from that autism research study.

Autism Research Results

After five months: Maternal Child Health Bureau research study

- Improved sleep and digestion
- Sensory problems improved by 38%, touch by 49%
- Parenting stress decreased by 44%
- Social skills increased and children were more affectionate
- Decreased aggression and behavior problems, fewer meltdowns
- Improved receptive language

After two years: Maternal Child Health Bureau research study

Improvements in touch:

- **Touch abnormalities** decreased to a mean normalization of 72%. This means that for all children, the average touch scores moved 72% of the distance from the original problems toward normal sensory scores. (50% of children with mild touch problems improved 100%.
- **Consistency**. Children whose parents correctly implemented all 12 QST movements daily (Full Fidelity) showed a full 87% change toward normalization of touch scores. 60% of children receiving QST with full fidelity achieved normal touch scores.

    Comparatively, the children receiving less than full fidelity showed a 61% change toward normalization, while only 24% of children achieved normal touch scores.

Improvements in Self-Regulation, Socialization and Language:

- **Self-Regulation** improved by 49%
- **Language** improved 54% in children on the mild end of the autism spectrum
- **Social**. Children participated more in family life and were more receptive to connecting with others.
- **In summary:** every child continued to improve. Progressive normalization of tactile responses was associated with progressive improvements of social skills, language and behavioral "self-regulation".

Improvements in severity of autism:

- **Overall** severity of autism reduced by 44%. 25% of all children in the study moved off the spectrum. (50% of children on the mild end moved off the spectrum).

Sadly, Louisa's next research project, the *QST Sensory Kids Pilot Study*, using the *QST Sensory Protocol* for the larger group of children who have challenges with sensory and self-regulation difficulties (though not on the autism spectrum), had to be discontinued due to her untimely death. Both the autism and sensory protocols use the same 12 QST movements; however, those movements were ordered in a different sequence that specifically addresses the developmental issues particular to each group. The *QST Sensory Protocol* was intentionally adapted to start with the 'making a connection' movement, a movement designed specifically to begin the treatment by engaging social connection between parent and child through the parent's attuned touch.

Important Research Takeaways for Sensory and Behavior Problems

What helps

1. **Be consistent.** To get the most out of QST, you must do it regularly. You don't have to do it perfectly, just do it!

    - With high frequency (5–7 nights per week), 50% of children on the mild end of the autism spectrum showed 100% normalization of touch abnormalities. Even 17% of children on the severe end showed normalization of touch.
    - Greater frequency per week also improved behavioral and self-regulation difficulties.
    - When daily frequency dropped, treatment results dropped in direct proportion. But the good news is that progress resumed when frequency increased again.

2. **Be patient.** Children with milder symptoms recovered faster.

- But even children with severe symptoms achieved normalization of scores over time.
- Parents who stayed with QST saw continued improvements at the end of one year and even more improvement at two years.

What you can expect

1. **Improvements in touch.** Parents who gave QST to even the most severely sensitive autistic children enjoyed a significant reduction in their children's touch abnormalities.
2. **Improved behavior and self-regulation.** Studies found real and cumulative improvements in social-emotional skills, language, behavior and self-regulation.
3. **Increased bonding and connection.** Studies confirmed what Louisa and every QST Therapist see every day, that all parents report an increase in bonding, affection and touch that is more related and connected by the end of the first year.

Dr. Silva's Published Research

The following is the list of studies published by Louisa Silva, MD, and her co-authors. Full reference citations and links to each of the studies can be found on the Qigong Sensory Training Institute website (www.QSTI.org/published-studies/).

QST Autism Protocol

- *QST massage for 6–12-year-olds with Autism Spectrum Disorder: An extension study.* (2016)
- *One and two-year outcomes of treating preschool children with autism with a Qigong massage protocol: An observational follow-along study.* (2016)
- *First skin biopsy reports in children with autism show loss of C-tactile fibers.* (2016)
- *About face: Evaluating and managing tactile impairment at the time of autism diagnosis.* (2015)
- *Early intervention with a parent-delivered massage protocol directed at tactile abnormalities decreases the severity of autism and improves child-to-parent interactions: A replication study.* (2015)
- *Treatment of tactile impairment in young children with autism: Results with Qigong massage.* (2013)
- *Prevalence and significance of abnormal tactile responses in young children with autism.* (2013)
- *Alternative support for families with autistic children in Lithuania.* (2012)
- *Qigong massage for motor skills in young children with Cerebral Palsy and Down Syndrome (2012)*
- *Early Intervention for autism with a parent-delivered Qigong massage program: A randomized controlled trial.* (2011)
- *Qigong massage treatment for sensory and self-regulation problems in young children with autism: A randomized controlled trial.* (2009)
- *A model and treatment for autism at the convergence of Chinese medicine and neuroscience: First 130 cases.* (2011)
- *Autism Parenting Stress Index: Initial psychometric evidence.* (2011)
- *Sense and Self-Regulation Checklist, a measure of comorbid autism symptoms: Initial psychometric evidence.* (2012)
- *Outcomes of a pilot training program in a Qigong massage intervention for young children with autism.* (2008)
- *Improvement in sensory impairment and social interaction in young children with autism following treatment with an original Qigong massage methodology.* (2007)
- *A medical Qigong methodology for Early Intervention in Autism Spectrum Disorder.* (2005)

QST Sensory Protocol - Down Syndrome and Cerebral Palsy studies

- *Improved speech following parent-delivered Qigong massage in young children with Down Syndrome: A pilot randomized controlled trial.* (2013)

QST research from independent researchers

- Tal-Atzili, O., & Salls, J. (2017, May 19). Qigong Sensory Training pilot study: A tactile home program for children with or at-risk for autism. *Journal of Occupational Therapy, Schools, & Early Intervention*, 10(4), 366–388. [https://doi.org/10.1080/19411243.2017.1325819]
- Jerger, K.K., Lundegard, L., Piepmeier, A., Faurot, K., Ruffino, A., Jerger, M., & Belger, A. (2018, April 5). Neural mechanisms of Qigong Sensory Training massage for children with Autism Spectrum Disorder: A feasibility study. *Global Advances in Health and Medicine*, 7, 2164956118769006. [https://doi.org/10.1177/2164956118769006]

Independent systematic reviews – American Occupational Therapy Association

The following three comprehensive systematic reviews are part of the American Occupational Therapy Association's evidence-based project and published in the *American Journal of Occupational Therapy.*

- Tanner, K., Schmidt, E., Martin, K., & Bassi, M. (2020). Interventions within the scope of occupational therapy practice to improve motor performance for children ages 0–5 years: A systematic review. *American Journal of Occupational Therapy*, 74, 7402180060p1–7402180060p40. [https://doi.org/10.5014/ajot.2020.039644]
- Kingsley, K., Sagester, G., & Weaver, L.L. (2020). Interventions supporting mental health and positive behavior in children ages birth–5 yr: A systematic review. *American Journal of Occupational Therapy*, 74, 7402180050. [https://doi.org/10.5014/ajot.2020.039768]
- Bodison, S.C., & Parham, L.D. (2018). Specific sensory techniques and sensory environmental modifications for children and youth with sensory integration difficulties: A systematic review. *American Journal of Occupational Therapy*, 72, 7201190040. [https://doi.org/10.5014/ajot.2018.029413]

Appendix H

Accessing Online QST Support Materials

To Access All Online Instructional Videos and QST Support Materials

Go to: Please go to https://resourcecentre.routledge.com/books/9781032419299

Scroll down: Scroll down to **Content** at the bottom of the page.

Complete question: To verify your purchase, please use your book to look up the answer to the question in box. Type the answer in the area provided, but BEFORE you click submit, be sure to . . .

Record your answer: First, write the answer here for future reference:
Answer to access question _____
You will need to use this answer and follow these same steps each time you want to access the videos or QST forms.

Ok . . . now click *Submit*: You now have access to the Videos and Support Materials. And, with this same answer, you have unlimited quick access whenever you want in the future.

Link to Support Materials Includes

- All Online Instructional Videos

- *QST Sensory Movement Chart*

- *Sensory and Self-Regulation Checklists: including Start Date, Mid-Year Check and Year-End Evaluations.*

- *Parent Stress Index: including Start Date, Mid-Year Check and Year-End Evaluation forms.*

- *Daily Routine Organizer Chart*

Index

Note: Page numbers in *italics* indicate figures and page numbers in **bold** indicate tables.

adapting touch in QST: Adrian's story 141–143; body language cues and 90–97; a mother's story 173–174, 182–183; pain and 135; reflections from a QST master trainer 141–143; for safety and calm 37

affective neuropathways 7

affective touch *see* touch, attuned

aggressive behavior: biting 107, 176; food allergies and 118; forms of 175; hitting 107, 176; kicking 107, 176; pinching 107, 176; sensory overload and **106**; simple technique to stop 175–176; spitting 107, 176; stress-mode and 18; survival-mode and 16, 107; technique to minimize 107–108; tone of parent voice and 107, 176

allergies *see* food allergies and intolerances

alternative treatments 8–9, 135

anxiety 15, 31, 38, 112, 186, 191

appease mode 18

appetite 112, 118, 205

appetite improvement 118

arching *see* back

arching during QST 79

arm movement during QST: arms and legs alternating 90; making a connection 66–67, 206

assertive behavior 187–188

attention: focusing 24, 65, 108, 180–181; self-regulation milestones 22, *23*, 24, 195; transitions and 108

attuned connection: calmness and 45; mother's story 182–183; safe boundaries and 42–45

attuned touch: brain and 26; parent emotions and 132; reciprocal 133–134; safety and 38; sensory language and 38; touch techniques and 63

attuning to body/behavioral cues 7–8, 19, 43, 50, 65, 153–154, 182–183

attuning to child's energy level 133–135

autism: language improvements and 170; QST Autism Protocol and 9, 210, 214–215; QST techniques and 3, 110, 126, 210, 217; research results 217–219; sense of touch and 35; sensory difficulties and 1, 214–215

Avis, Ra 42

awareness: attuned touch and 133, 162; emotions and 190; in fingers 140, 170; neural networks and 27; self-awareness and 37–38, 187; sensory 14, 41; of skin 63, 128; slowing down 42; touch and 27; *see also* body-awareness

back: arching during QST 79, 91, 153–154; movement during QST 145; no sensation in 128

bad days, help with 145

Baeyens, Sabine 177

balance: body and behavioral cues 43; boundaries and 42–46; communicating 45; connection and 42–46; parent-child relationship and 41; sensory messages and 45–46

Baniel, A. 42

behavior: aggression and 18, **106**; assertive 187–188; doing the opposite **106**; fight or flight reaction 18, 175; immature sensory nervous system and 4, 13, 105; a mother's story 173–174; not listening **106**; reframing bad 1, 14, 98, 182; refusing to cooperate **106**; rejection and 18; research results 218–219; running away **106**; self-regulation problems and 103–105; sensory problems

and 3–4, 134; signs of progress 205; stress-mode and 17–18; willfulness 18
belly: Chinese medicine perspective 152; discomfort 91; distended 118; fear and 152, 185; opening and strengthening flow to 152; signs QST is working 171; strong emotions and 152; support hands and 145–146
Belly Circles movement 73–74, 145
Bergeron, Rosimery 195
bicycle adaptation to movement 87, 96
biting 107, 175–176
bloating 118
blocks: belly discomfort and 92, 99; ears and 81, 92; energy flow and 7, 63, 94–95, 101, 115; hand gestures and 93–94; head and 76, 99, 101; hyper after QST 94; layers 92, 149; ribs and 95–96
body and behavioral cues during QST: arms and legs alternating 90; attuning to 7–8, 19, 43, 50, 65, 153–154; back arching 79, 91; balance and 42–43; belly discomfort 91; burping 91; Chinese medicine perspective 35–36; connection and 42, 45, 138; coughing 91; discomfort 91; ear discomfort 91–92; emotional releases 92; eye contact 138; eye rubbing 93; family helpers and 145; feet sensitive/painful 93; fingers painful/ticklish 93; hand gestures 93–94; humming and 80, 94, 138; hyperactivity and 94; jumping up 94; just right touch and 90; leg movements 79, 94–95; lips move 95, 139; non-verbal 26; pain 91; quick reference chart for **96**; reading 153–154; ribs stiff/tight 95–96; smiling and 138; ticklishness 79, 93, 96; tongue moves 139; yawning 96
body-awareness: energy flow and 179–180; motor skills and 30–31; QST techniques and 170; safety and 177; touch and 30–31
body-brain connection 31
body language during QST: attuning to 56; child 56; important cues to look for 90–97; just right touch and 90; parents and 90, 97; *see also* body and behavioral cues during QST
body map: brain and 37; self-awareness and 37–38; sensory signals and 37; tactile communication and 7; touch signals and 30
boundaries: assertive behavior and 187–188; balance and 42–43, 46; connection and 45; organizing 41–46; setting safe 41–42, 43–46, 187–189
bowel movements 114–115, 138, 152

brain: body map and 37; mode **18**; points that help 178–179; skin-brain connections 29–30, 137–138; somatosensory area of 30; touch signals and 26–27, 29–30, 37, 138, 140
breathing exercise: for rest-relax-relate response 132
Broderick, Maria 154
burping 91

calm: attuning to child's energy level 133–135; calming movements 50; calm-listening mode 13; connection and 33, 38, 42, 45; lending your 132–133; need for during QST 56; parents and 37, 56, 65, 143, 145; sensory responses and 2; stress and 50
calm-listening mode 13
Cascio, C.J. 28
catch-up development 172
cerebral palsy 220
challenging behaviors: aggressive behavior 107–108; behavioral self-regulation problems and 103–105; causes of 103–105; communication difficulties 103–104; lack of skills/maturation 103–104; physical problems and 103–104; planting/sitting 109; QST skills for 105, 107; quick reference chart for **106**; stress and 103–105, **106**, 110–111; transitions and 108
changes during QST: body cues and 138–139; emotional releases and 92; marking progress 161–165, 169–174; setting goals for 57
chemicals: absorbed through skin 116–117; breathing in 116; in environment 116–117; in foods 116, 152
chest: energy flow and 151; relaxing 145, 150–152, 171, 185; signs QST is working 171; support hands and 145–146
Chinese medicine: daily energy cycle and 119; diet and nutrition in 112; Eastern perspective on sensory difficulties 35–36; energy flow and 7–8, 91, 148–149, 178–181; on fear 152; points that help the brain 178–179; QST techniques and 2–3, 143; reading body and behavioral cues 153–154; strong emotions and 152; therapeutic model and 7
circulation: Chinese medicine perspective 2; elimination of toxins and 117, 143; pain and lack of 93; patting and 64; QST movements and 65–66, 72, 75; ticklishness and lack of 75, 96
Clayton, Sue xviii, 148

clinicians and professionals: clinical method and 8–9; professional certification in QST methods 9; QST techniques and 6–9
commitment to daily routine 120
communication: balance and 45–46; gestural language and 140–141, 170; non-verbal 31–32, 41; parent touch and 39; sensory language and 35; touch as 31–32, 39
communication difficulties: challenging behaviors and 103–104; language of touch and 32; not listening **106**
connection: attuned 42–43; balance and 42–46; body and 42, 45, 138; body-brain 31; calm-to-calm 33, 38, 42, 45; heart-to-heart 32–33, 38, 132; intention-to-intention 33; safe organizing boundaries and 41–42, 43–45; skin-brain 29–30, 137–138; social 30, 68–70, 191–192, 195; support hands and 145; technique for social 7, 68, 71, 191–192; touch-brain 26–27, 29–30, 37, 138; *see also* body-brain connection; heart-to-heart connection; touch-brain connection; touch-face-heart connection
constipation 73, 112, 115, 152, 205
contraindications to QST 210
control: controlling fours and 126, 188–189; need for 187–189; parent guilt and 189; predictability and 188–189; reframing 188–189; of routines 158; self-control 25, 147, 189
controlling fours 126, 188–189
co-regulation: co-piloting 38; co-regulating circuit 38; interbrain and 38–39, 41; non-verbal communication and 38; self-regulation and 37–38; social connections and 195; *see also* touch co-regulation
Costa, Gerard xvii-xviii, 50
coughing 91
Crohn's disease 193
C-tactile nerve fibers: pleasurable touch and 29–30; touch-fiber highway 7, 29–30, 36–37

daily routine organizer **121**
daily routines: bedtime and 194; four risk periods for dropping 156–157; importance of rhythmic 119–120; ingraining QST in 158
deep relaxation 150
defense-mode 175, 177; *see also* survival-mode
development: digestive health and 112; emotional 31–32; first year 21–22; immature sensory nervous system and 13; motor skills and 30,

66, 75, 79–80, 85, 171; opening roadblocks to 140–141; oversensitivity to touch and 141; regression and 189–191; touch and 27–28, 32; *see also* pyramid of learning
diarrhea 73, 112, 114, 152, 205
diet and nutrition: avoiding artificial food color and flavor 114, 160; avoiding milk products 114, 118; avoiding processed foods 114, 116, 152, 159; avoiding toxins 115–116; Chinese medicine perspective 112; digestion and 75; food choices 113–114; food intolerances and allergies 114; gluten-free 118; healthy development and 112–113; hyperactivity and 113, 160; importance of home cooked food 114, 116, 152, 160; rhythmic daily routines and 119; warm and cooked food 113, 152; *see also* food
digestion: difficulties 75, 112, 114–115; energy and 113; immature sensory nervous system and 112; regulating 152; self-regulation and 113; self-regulation milestones 22, *23*, 24; signs of progress 203; warm and cooked food 113, 152
direction of QST movements: clockwise/counterclockwise 73, 91, 93–95, 145; strokes down body 64, 66, 71–72, 75–81
directions: doing the opposite **106**; teaching simple 109–110
discomfort during QST: blocks in energy flow 148; body cues and 91–92; pain and ticklishness 135–136; parent unawareness of 43–45; patting and pressing 135, 145; touch alternatives and 9, 135
distracting 31, 44, 57
distraction: learning to ignore 147; as tool during QST 134; transitions and 181–182; videos and 132
dog days 155–156
Down Syndrome 210, 217, 220
Down the Back: one hand movement 77–78; two hand movement 79–80
Down the Legs movement 75
Down the Sides movement 82–83, 150

early intervention: autism and 214–215; family-centered approaches 214; QST and 5, 133, 214–216
Early Self-Regulation Milestones: appetite and digestion 22, *23*, 24; being soothed/self-soothing 22, *23*, 24–25; developmental steps and 4; orientation and attention 22, *23*, 24; sleep and 22, *23*, 24

ears: blocked 79, 92, 114; clearing 145; discomfort during QST 37, 91–92; empty 91–92; Extra Clearing movement 81; listening problems 140, 149–150; patting and pressing 150; sensitivity to touch 140; signs QST is working 170; support hands and 145
Ear to Hand movement 84, 150
easy button 179–180
Elliott, Matt xviii
emotional regulation: problems with 125; QST to support 147–148; social touch and 28
emotional releases 72, 92, 152, 183–185
emotions: belly and 152; children and 25, 30–31, 37, 72, 74, 92; Chinese medicine perspective 152; emotional development 31; expressed during QST 183–184; getting through hard times 185–186; a mother's story 182–183; parents and 43, 47–48, 50–52, 56, 132; parent touch and 31, 132; regression and 190; release of emotional bubbles 152, 183–185; self-regulation and 195; stress and 50–52; stuck inside 31; *see also* parent emotions
empathy 32, 134, 137
emptiness 91–92, 96
energy: attuning to child's 133–135, 141; daily flow 119; daily routines and 120; digestion and 113; doing QST 55; emptiness and 91–92; energy blocks 63; head and 148–149, 178; movement in body 153–154; optimizing daily 119; parent intention and 65; Qi and 7; sleep and 148; *see also* parent energy; Qi
energy flow: attuning to bring calm 133; Chinese medicine perspective 7–8, 91, 148, 153–154, 178–181; ear discomfort and blocked 91–92; opening to resolve tantrums 150–152; optimizing daily 119; regulating digestion and elimination 152; sleep problems and 148–149; throughout body 178–180
Extra Ear Clearing movement 81
Extra Neck Clearing movement 76, 149
eyes: avoids contact 68, 109; blinking/rubbing 93, 138; closing 138; making eye contact 17, 19, 24, 31, 69, 110, 130, 138; signs QST is working 139; twitching/fluttering 139

face-me-button 180–181
facial expression: children and 17, **18**, 109; parents and 19, 68, 107, 176; signs QST is working 139, 151; stress-mode and 17, **18**

family support teams 55–56
fast-acting nerve fibers 29–30
fear: belly and 152, 185; children and 15, 25, 31–32, 185; Chinese medicine perspective 152; fearful agitation 100; parents and 51, 100; during QST 92, 100
feet: energy in 178; heels drift up during QST 81, 96; pain and 93; sensitive to touch 93; signs QST is working 171; *see also* toes
fight-flight-or-freeze mode: behavior and 18, 175; defense-mode and 177; resistance to QST 98–99, 131; sensitivity to touch and 140; sensory problems and 16–17
fine motor development 66, 86
fingers: gestural language and 140–141, 170; normalizing sensitivity in 85, 140–141; pain and 135; pointing and 140, 170; signs QST is working 170; support hands and 145; ticklishness and 93, 135
Fingers movement 85
focus: attention and 24, 65, 108, 180–181; body cues and 49–50; breathing and 71; help with 50
food: avoiding artificial food color and flavor 114, 160; avoiding milk products 114, 118; avoiding processed 114, 116, 152, 159; difficulty digesting 114–115; eating narrow range of 112, 159; importance of home cooked 114, 116, 152, 160; ingestion of toxins from 115–116; intolerances and allergies 114, 117–118; nutritious choices 113–114; picky eating and 21, 58, 133, 139, 141, 173; preparation rules 113; toleration of textures in 140, 159; warmed and cooked 113, 152; *see also* appetite; diet and nutrition; digestion
food allergies and intolerances 114, 117–118
freeze mode 16–18, **18**, 19, 30, 56, 109, 140, 149
freeze response 16–18
frequency of QST: 6–7 vs. 3–4 days 56, 172–173; staying consistent 56, 155–160, 172–173
frustration: aggressive behavior and 107, 175–176; deep relaxation and 150; dog days and 155–156; parents and 17, 44–45, 47, 65, 100, 108, 133, 177, 181, 182–183; persisting through 141–143; self-soothing and 147

Garofallou, Linda 1, 3
Garofallou, Jim xix
gestural language 140–141, 170

getting help 57, 156, 211

getting started: keys to success 56–57; lessons from a mother 129–130; setting up 55–56

gluten-free, casein-free diet (GFCF) 118; *see also* diet and nutrition

goals: mid-year check-in 169; personal 57, 212; QST techniques and 144, 215; setting 57; start date 57; support groups and 212

gross motor development 78, 80, 171

growth spurts 170, 189, 193

gut microbiome 112

haircuts 142, 172

hand gestures 93–94

hand pressure and shape *see* touch

hands: aggressive behavior and 107, 176; helping hands and 144–146; poor awareness in 170; pushing away 94, 135; during QST 94; QST techniques 64–65, 100, 129; quieting 99

Harvey, Adrienne 158

head: down during QST 170; energy in 148–149, 178; laying down during QST 77–80; signs QST is working 170; starting position 82, 82

hearing: congested ears and 81, 114; listening problems 150; sensory overload and 98; in stress mode 17, 49, 140; tone of parent voice 17, 19; *see also* ears

heart-to-heart connection: QST techniques and 38, 132; touch and 32–33

hitting 44, 107, 133, 159, 175–176

Hopkins, Susan xix, 17

hormones: cascading 17; feel good 31; stress 17–18, 104, 109–110

humming 80, 94, 138

hyperactivity: artificial food coloring and flavors 160; clearing/tapping 142; following QST 94; gut microbiome and 112; importance of diet **106**, 112, 160; toxins and 117, 160

illness 115, 190

immature sensory nervous system: behavioral problems and 4, 13, 105; causes of 14–15; chemical burden in food and 116; digestion and 112; immature driver metaphor 37; inability to make transitions 181; over-reactivity and 15, 36; parent's touch and 4, 29–30; sensory overload and 13–15, 21; stress-mode and 17

inner abilities: be soothed to 24–25; self-regulation and 22, 36–38; self-soothing 22, 24–25, 31; shifting to calm 21–22, 36; shifting to safety 36

integration of movements: following QST 88, 184, 189; during QST 71, 88, 95, 136–139, 145–146

intention 6, 8, 33, 38–39, 42, 65; *see also* parents

interbrain: co-regulation and 38–39, 41; as wireless BlueTooth 38–39

interoception 14, 27

jumping up during QST 94, 183

kicking 44, 95, 107, 153–154, 175–176

knees: bending up during QST 78, 95, 145; kicking and 107, 176

language: gestural 140–141, 170; signs of progress 205; of touch 2, 32; *see also* communication; sensory language

learning ability: delays in 21; self-regulation and 175; sensory impairments and 30, 36; touch and 27, *28*

legs: floating/drawing up 95; kicking 95; movement during QST 90, 94–95, 145; relaxing 145

Lessons Learned from QST Autism Research 217–220

life changes 190

lips move during QST 93, 140–141

listening: calm-listening mode 13, 17; language of touch and 32; not listening **106**; opening the ears 149–150; problems with 149–150; refusal and 140; touch and 38–39, 140

love 1, 38, 43, 63, 132, 145, 186

lungs 95

lying down for QST 94, 99, 131, 170

Making a Connection 66

measuring progress: child's progress 58; daily QST routine and 57–58; Parenting Stress Index 59; parent progress 59; QST Progress Chart 58, *59*; Sense and Self-Regulation Checklist 58–61; *see also* Parenting Stress Index; QST Progress Chart; Sensory and Self-Regulation Checklist

medication 210

meltdowns: co-regulation and 38; emotional stress and 50–51; immature sensory nervous system and 15; naps to prevent 120; relaxation response and 151; rhythmic daily routines and 119; sensory overload and 13, 15, 25; *see also* tantrums

microbiome 112

mind: think-problem-solving 13

mindsight 49, 51
mini QST 110
misbehaving 14
motor skills: body awareness and 30–31; fine motor development 66, 83; gross motor development 78, 80, 171; legs and 75; parent touch and 31
movement chart *see* QST Sensory Movement Chart
movements: common questions related to 100–102; order of 50, 65–66, 90; patting and pressing 63–65; purpose of 63–64; troubleshooting 206–209
mucus congestion 114–115
Mulrooney, Kathy xix

nail trimming 150, 172
Neck, Extra Clearing movement 76, 149
need for control: assertive behavior and 187–188; controlling fours and 126, 188–189; predictability and 188–189; reframing 188–189
nerve fibers: fast-acting 29–30; peripheral 35; slow-acting 29; *see also* C-tactile nerve fibers
nervous system: autonomic 14, 71; basic neural networks 27; C-tactile nerve fibers 7, 29; development of 29, 195; down-regulating 43, 50–51, 98, 109; fast-acting fibers 29–30; maturation of 14; peripheral nerves and 35; relaxation response 49; self-regulation and 195; sensory difficulties and 1, 35; stress response 4, 48; sympathetic 25; touch-based interventions and 192; *see also* appease mode; calm-listening mode; fight-flight-or-freeze mode; immature sensory nervous system; shut-down mode; stress-mode
neural patterns: new 42
neurotransmitters, from gut microbiome 112
night terrors 186
non-verbal communication: autistic children and 215; body language and 18; children and 32, 107, 170, 176, 215; co-regulation and 38; eye contact and 31; parent touch and 8, 31–32, 39, 41, 133; sensory language and 41
noticing changes: mid-year check-in 161–165; progress over time 161; what they mean 170–171
Nourish and Integrate movement 88–89

numbness 136–137
nutrition *see* diet and nutrition

organizing patterns 126
optimizing daily energy 119–120
optional movements: Extra Ear Clearing movement 81; Extra Neck Clearing movement 76–80; Up-Up-Up movement 68–70
oversensitivity to touch: development and 140–141; pain and 135; pressing and 127; sensory triggers and 15–17; ticklishness and 135–136
overwhelmed feelings: communication difficulties and 104; immature sensory nervous system and 14–15; parents and 6, 48, 50–51, 100; planting/refusal to move 109; reactivity and 16; sensory overload and 14, 36, 45, 99; stress mode and 18; survival-mode and 16–17; touch and 32

pain: feet and 93; hypersensitivity 44; insensitivity to 157; lack of circulation and 93; during QST 91, 135–136; resistance to QST and 135; toes and 135, 186
parent-child relationship: balance and 41; QST theory and 7–8; safe boundaries and 41–42; touch and 7
parent emotions 43, 47–48, 50–52, 56, 132
parent energy: de-stressing and 50; doing QST 55, 57, 91–93, 134; low 148; patting movements and 64; self-regulation and 147; shape of hand and 63–64
Parenting Stress Index: mid-year check-in 162–163, *168*; start date 59, 162; year-end evaluations 196–197, *197*, 215
parents: agitation 48, 133; becoming overwhelmed 156; coaching and support for 156; creating support groups 212–213; emotions 43, 47–48, 50–52, 56, 132; energy and 50, 55, 57, 63–64, 91, 93, 147–148; fear and 51, 100; intention 6, 8, 33, 38–39, 42, 65; reading body cues 90, 97; self-care and 128–129, 182–183; self-compassion and 128–129; self-regulation and 4–5, 22, 25, 47–52; sense of calm and 37, 56, 65, 143, 145; skeptical 159; stress and 48–51; stress levels and 59, 170, 197, 215; support groups and 193, 212–213; support hands 89; touch and 1–2, 27, 132; voice and 176; *see also* quieting emotional stress; quieting physical stress

parent touch: attuning to child's energy level 133–135, 141; communication and 39; emotions and 31; lack of sensitivity and 210; non-verbal communication and 8, 31–32, 39, 41, 133; parent-child relationship and 7; primacy of 7; safety and 176, 195; sensory growth and 4; sensory language and 30, 35–38

patting and pressing: discomfort during QST 37; energy blocks and 63; over-sensitivity and 127; patting movements 64; pressing movements 64; repetitions 64–65; sensory language and 37–38; sensory problems and 35; shape of hand 63; slowing down 42; switching between 101; under-sensitivity and 63, 128; weekly letters and 127–128

pause/pausing 42, 48–49, 51, 65, 161

Perry, Bruce D. 30

pinching 107, 175–176

planting/refusal to move **106**, 109

pointing 140, 170

Poling, Linda xviii

Porges, Stephen 195

potty training 139, 174

predictability 188–189

preparation for QST 76, 81

preschool: doing better in 14, 142; environmental toxins and 117; homemade snacks and 116; over-reactivity and 15

pressing movements 64, 127; see also patting and pressing

progress: checking in on goals 169; leveling off of 157; mid-year check-in 161–165; a mother's story 171–172; noticing changes 161–165; signs of 155–156, 205; start date 162–165; year-end evaluations 198

proprioception 14, 27

Pyramid of Learning 28

Qi: channels in child's body 115; defined 7; parent energy flow and 64, 148; self-regulation and 148

Qigong Sensory Training (QST): contraindications to 210; defined 2; parents and 6, 143; professional certification in 7, 9, 214; QSTI 9, 156, 211, 219; QST trainers 58, 156, 210–211, 216; research results 6, 215–220; sensory experiences and 1

Qigong Sensory Training Institute (QSTI) 9, 156, 211, 219

QST see Qigong Sensory Training (QST)

QST Autism Protocol 9, 210, 214–215, 217, 219

QST Down Syndrome Protocol 210, 217, 220

QST movements: benefits of 143–144; Chinese medical healing and 2; grandmothers and cultural tradition of 27–28; unusual taste during 144; see also direction of QST movements; integration of movement

QST Online Support: accessing materials 221; getting personalized help 211

QST Parent Support Facebook page 202, 211

QST Progress Chart 58, 59; mid-year check-in 162–163, 163, 164, 164; start date 59, 162–165; year-end evaluations 198, 197

QST routine: building trust and 38; consistency and 42, 56; daily practice and 5–6, 19; dog days 155–156; family support teams and 55–56; four risk periods for dropping 156–157; getting help 57; getting started 55–59; measuring progress 57–61; rhythmic touch and 27; sensory language and 2; setting goals 57; staying consistent 56, 155–160, 172–173; time of day 55

QST Sensory Kids Pilot Study 218

QST Sensory Movement Chart 5, 204; important signs of progress 205; support groups and 212–213; what the twelve movements do 203

QST Sensory Protocol 217–218, 220

QST techniques: for aggression 107–108; autism and 3, 110, 126, 210, 217; for clinicians and professionals 6–9; daily routine and 5; early intervention and 133, 214–216; easy button 179–180; to encourage conversation 32, 181; everyday skills 109–110; extra 175–186; face-me-button 180–181; family helpers and 144; getting out of defense mode 177; getting personalized help 211; mini QST 110; parent questions on 100–102; for tantrums 194; for transitions 108

QST touch techniques: attuned touch 56–57; challenging behaviors and 103; parent training 142; patting and pressing 63–65, 101; sensory language and 37–38; see also patting and pressing

quieting emotional stress 50–52

quieting physical stress 48–50

reactions during QST see body and behavioral cues during QST

ready to learn 171–172

red dye 115–116, 160

reflux 152
regression 189–191
regulation: ability to be soothed/self-soothing
22, *23*, 24–25; of appetite and digestion
22, *23*, 24; of focus 22, 24; of orientation
and attention 22, *23*, 24; regulatory/
organizational process 7, 37; of sleep 22, *23*,
24; *see also* self-regulation
rejection: of parent's touch 27; soothing and 38;
stress-mode and 18
relaxation during QST: children and 84, 95, 127,
138, 150–152, 175, 184–185, 203; deep
relaxation and 150; parents and 132, 134;
see also self-soothing
Relax Chest movement 71–72, 150–152, 185
Relax Legs movement 86
relax-relate mode: defense against stress 18–19,
36; development of 25; survival-mode and
175; touch techniques and 145
repetitions of QST movements: internal guidance
and 38; organizing boundaries and 42;
patting and pressing 64–65; repetitive
rhythmic input 30; sensory language
and 41
resilience 15, 25–26
resistance to QST: avoidance without agitation
99; common questions related to 100–102;
discomfort and 45; doing the opposite 13,
19; fearful agitation 100; fight or flight
reaction 98–99, 131; pain and 135; parent
response to 56–57, 131; refusal to lie down
99; ticklishness and 135; in toddlers 100,
133–135; working with 131–132; *see also*
planting/refusal to move
rest following QST 88–89
restraint: care activities and 133; never using
98–100, 131, 144
rhythm: interbrain and 38; language of touch and
32; pressing movements and 64; safety and
30; structure and 5, 121; touch and 27, 41
rhythmic daily routines 5, 19, 27, 43, 119
rhythmic wave 145–146
ribs, stiff/tight 95–96, 151
risk periods for stopping QST 156–157
rubbing eyes 110, 138, 181, 206

safety: attuned touch and 38; body and 177; parent
voice and touch 176, 195; of social contact
30; support hands and 145–146
school behavior: environmental toxins and 117;
food additives and 160; self-regulation and

21; sensory problems and 44, 159, 190, 192;
social skills and 44
scientific studies *see* Lessons learned from QST
Autism Research
seizures 210
self-awareness 37–38, 187
self-care: parents and 128–129, 182–183; weekly
letters and 128–129; *see also* parents
self-compassion 128–129
self-control 147, 189
self-regulation: behavioral problems and 4,
103–105; co-regulation and 37–38;
digestion and 113; emotions and 147–148;
importance of 147, 195; inner capacity
for 36–37; in later life 195; milestones in
21–22, *23*, 24–25, 195; nervous system and
195; organizing boundaries 43; parents and
4–5, 22, 25, 46, 48–52, 147; restoring 26;
self-control and 147; sensory problems and
4, 19, 25; sleep and 113, 148–149; stress
and 48–52; tactile communication and 8;
see also Early Self-Regulation Milestones
self-soothing: self-regulation milestones 22,
23, 24–25, 195; signs of 138; transitions
and 182
sense of safety *see* safety
sense of self 30, 32, 42, 157, 187
senses: eight basic 14; hearing and 192; opening
up with QST 144; touch and development of
27, 192; vision and 192
Sensory and Self-Regulation Checklist: form for
60–61; measuring progress 58–59; mid-
year check-in 162–163, *166–167*; start date
58–59, 162; year-end evaluations 196–198,
199–200
sensory doors 36
sensory language: attuned touch and 38; non-
verbal communication and 41; parent
touch and 35–38; patting and pressing 37;
QST routine and 2, 35–38; responses to
children 41, 43; self-regulation and 4; tactile
communication and 7, 35, 37; *see also* body
language during QST
sensory messages: balance and 45–46; organized
7, 21, 36, 41; parent touch and 30
sensory overload: behavioral problems and
13–14; hearing and 98; immature sensory
nervous system and 13–15, 21; meltdowns
and 13, 15, 25; survival-mode and 36
sensory problems: autism and 1; behavioral
problems and 3–4, 134; changing

perspective 1, 35–36; energy blocks and 149; fight-flight-or-freeze mode 16–17; interfering with school 44–45, 192–193; normalizing responses 2; patting and pressing 35, 127; research results 218–219; self-regulation and 4, 19, 25; survival-mode and 13–14; tactile communication and 7

sensory solution 19

sensory system: at birth 14; causes of challenging behaviors 103–105; causes of immature 13–15; immature 2, 13–15, 21, 30, 36, 105; oversensitivity and 135; sensory triggers and 15–16; signs of progress 205; *see also* immature sensory nervous system

sensory triggers: aggression and 107, 175; emotional releases and 92; fight-or-flight response 94, 98–99, 131, 175; immature sensory responses and 15; Morse code 37; over-reactivity and 4, 15–17, 29, 36; rapid 15–16; self-soothing and 108, 110; slow 15–16; survival-mode and 4, 16; under-reactivity and 36

setting up 55–56

settling down 101, 148, 172, 179, 186

Shanker, S. xix, 14, 103

shoes and socks 93

shoulders: relaxing muscles in 65, 149; sleep and 149; tense/lifted 48–49, 82–83, 110, 149, 186

shut-down mode 16–17, 181

siblings 191–192

Siegel, Daniel 49, 51

signs QST is working 137–139, 170–171

Silva, Louisa 1–3, 5, *23*, 35, 39, 130, 193, 214, 217, 219

skeptical parents 159

skin: awareness of 63; boundary and 42; chemicals absorbed through 116–117; as external nervous system 29; patting and pressing 63–64, 75, 128; sensitivity to touch 75, 80, 93, 135–136; sensory nerves in 1, 29–31, 35–36, 127, 137; touch-brain connection and 29

skin-brain connections 29–30, 137–138

skin-to-skin contact 195

sleep: energy flow and 148–149; following QST 142, 149; importance of 119–120, 148; problems with 147, 149; self-regulation and 113, 148–149; self-regulation milestones 22, *23*, 24; signs of progress 205

slow-acting nerve fibers 29

slowness, focused 42

smell: chemicals and 116; during QST 143; release of toxins 117; sense of 14, 44, 148, 174, 192

smelly poops 117

smiling 138, 170

social circles 191–192

social connections/interactions: attuned touch and 218; co-regulation and 195; pleasurable touch and 30; safety and 19, 30; self-regulation and 22, 141; Up-Up-Up movement 68–70, 192; widening social circles 191–192

social development 170

social skills 44, 57, 139, 147, 205

social touch 28

soft eyes 17

soft spot 79, 82, 178

somatosensory area 30

special needs: QST for 187–195; support groups and 193

speech 85, 135, 140

spitting 107, 175–176

stress: being a detective 103–105; calming 50; challenging behaviors and 103–105, **106**, 110–111; easy button and 179–180; exercises for 49–51; first line of defense against 18, 22; good vs. bad 110–111; hormones 17; nervous system response to 4, 17, 48; parents and 48–51; quieting emotional 50–52; quieting physical 48–50; self-regulation and 48–52; terrible twos and 187

stress behavior 105, 175–176, 187–188

stress-mode: behavior and 17–18; body language and 17–18, **18**; facial expressions and 17, **18**; fight-flight-or-freeze mode 17, 98–99; need for control and 187–189; tone of parent voice 99

stuck in stress mode 126, 187–188

success: hints to best results 64–65; keys to 56–57; noticing changes 161–162; reviewing progress 155–156; in school 192–193

support groups 193, 212–213

support hands 145–146

survival-mode: aggressive behavior and 107; appease mode and 18; behavior and 18; communication during 17; fight or flight reaction 98–99; freeze response and 18; relax-relate mode 18–19, 175; sensory overload and 36; sensory problems and 13–14; sensory triggers and 4, 16–17, 27, 36 tactile communication: clinical method and 8–9; primacy of touch and 7; self-regulation and 8; sensory language and 7–8; *see also* C-tactile nerve fibers

Tal-Atzili, Orit 133, 141–143, 214–216

tantrums: emotional stress and 50; need for control 188–189; opening energy flow 150–152; QST techniques and 194; relaxation response and 151; self-regulation and 22; sensory overload and 13, 15; stress and **106**; *see also* meltdowns

taste: sense of 14, 148, 192; unusual during QST 143

teachers 21, 44, 164, 202

terrible twos 117, 126, 187–188; *see also* need for control

ticklishness: fingers and 93; lack of circulation and 75, 96; pressing movements for 75, 77, 79, 82, 93; sensitivity to touch 135–136; toes and 87, 96

tiptoe, walking on 80, 141, 179, 203

toes: painful 135, 186; sensitivity to touch 93, 135; support hands and 145; ticklishness and 87, 96, 136

Toes movement 87

toilet training *see* potty training

tone of parent voice: aggressive behavior and 107, 176; calm and 41, 99, 109; hearing in stress mode 17, 19, 107; heart-to-heart connection and 33; simple directions and 110; stress and 49

tongue 139–140

tooth brushing 142

touch: adapting 37; affective 7–9; attuned 19, 26–27, 48, 132–135; body awareness and 30–31; brain and 26–27, 29–30, 37; communication and 31–32, 39; co-regulation 8, 14, 24–25, 38; cultural tradition of 27–28; emotional development and 31, 132; essential to life 28; heart-to-heart connection and 32–33; hyper/over-sensitivity to 15–17, 107, 127, 135–136, 139; just right 90; like food for brain 30; listening through 39; non-verbal communication 31–32; paradox of 8; pleasurable 29–30; resistance to 131; senses and 27, 192; sensory language and 2, 7, 32,

35, 37; signals to brain 27; shape of hand 63; under-sensitivity to 63, 128, 139; *see also* parent touch

touch-brain connection: guided touch and 26; normalizing sensitivity in fingers 140; signs QST is working 139; skin and 29, 138; touch signals and 27, 29–30, 37

touch-face-heart connection 19

tough spots, don't skip 56–57

toxins: behavioral reactions and 117; detoxing and 193; diet and 115–116, 160; digestion problems and 115; elimination of 117, 148; exposure via breathing chemicals 116; exposure via ingestion 115–116; exposure via skin absorption 116–117; food allergies and intolerances 117–118; hyperactivity and 117, 160; markers and 117; regression and 190

transitions: difficulty with **106**, 108, 181–182; immature sensory nervous system and 181; QST routine and 142, 151; techniques for 181–182

trauma 15, 43, 72, 174, 186, 188

Troubleshooting Guide 206–209

under-sensitivity to touch: challenging behaviors and 157; development and 139; patting and 63, 128

Up-Up-Up Movement for Social Connection 68–70, 192

verbal communication: adapting responses 41; on aggressive behavior 107, 176; improvements in 215; simple directions and 110; on touch 127

vestibular system 27

wandering off **106**

weekly letters: for daily regulation 147–153; extra techniques 175–186; getting the most out of 125–126; introduction 125; key issues and 5; marking progress 161–174; mastering the basics 127–146; QST for special needs 187–195; staying consistent 155–160; year-end evaluations 196–198, 202

yawning 96, 138

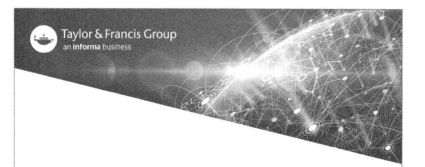